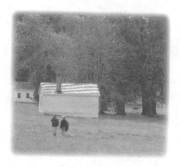

# May I Walk You Home?

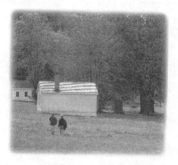

*courage and comfort for
caregivers of the very ill*

stories by  JOYCE HUTCHISON
prayers by  JOYCE RUPP

**ave maria press**
Notre Dame, Indiana

First Printing: January, 1999
Second Printing: July, 1999
29,000 copies in print

---

International Standard Book Number: 0-87793-670-6

Cover and text design by Katherine Robinson Coleman

Printed and bound in the United States of America.

To Gary,

my husband of thirty-two years

and

my friend forever,

who encouraged me to write these stories

about my patients and families

before this book was ever a dream of mine.

—JOYCE HUTCHISON

To my uncle Ivan Rupp,

his life and death

were my great teachers,

and to my aunt Jean,

her loving care of Ivan

inspired and blessed my life.

—JOYCE RUPP

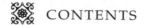 CONTENTS

## THE STORIES

# THE STORIES

My husband, Gary, was always so supportive of my work and never begrudged the long hours when it took me away from home. He would often tell me when I came home late that if I helped someone who was struggling that it was worth the sacrifice to him. Gary, perhaps you had so much understanding and compassion because of the journey you were traveling. Even though I had not completed these stories before you died, I have constantly felt your little nudge from afar. Thank you, Gary, for your faithful love and support.

I would never have co-authored this book without the expertise of Joyce Rupp, who has written many excellent, inspiring books. She was always there with her knowledge, supportive friendship, and unconditional love. Thank you, Joyce, for continually guiding me on my spiritual journey by your presence in my life.

To my children Joe, Mike, and Julie, I give thanks and love for the wonderful human beings that you have become.

To Dr. Buroker, thanks for teaching me so much about the care and concern for patients and families at the time of a life threatening diagnosis and treatment. Your upbeat manner fostered hope. Everyone you care for feels that they are very special to you and I believe that happens because you give so much of yourself to them.

To Dr. Sara Scott and Dr. Tim Vermillion for their dedication to the dying patients and their families, and for their openness to whoever or whatever that patient was about. You both conveyed great respect for each person that you came in contact with on that final journey. Thank you both for the great inspiration you were to me.

Thank you Lynne Kinseth for the never-ending support that you give to the dying patients and their families. Your sensitivity and intense interest in those folks is a wonderful blessing to them, as it is freely given and is truly genuine.

I want to acknowledge two very special women, Connie McCreery and Alice Wegner, Home Health Aides, who take care of their patients as if they are their own family. You both are a great blessing to the patients that you care for as you go the extra mile to make their days and hours the best that they can be.

I am grateful to Faye Petersen and Linda Carey, coworkers. They taught me so much of what I am about and did so with affirmation and love. We shared a mutual love for our hospice patients and families and this common bond was the beginning of a valued friendship.

Thank you to all my widow friends (the Ssenippah group) for the friendship, support, fun, and mutual experience that we have shared on our journey. As we were forming our group of support during a time of pain and loneliness we learned that we could laugh and love again and, therefore, "Ssenippah" (happiness spelled backwards) became our name.

Martha Kraber is a very valuable presence on my

journey of life. She quietly loves those she comes in contact with and is the sister I never had. Thanks, Martha.

A very special thank you to Sister Eve Kavanagh for introducing Gary and me to the ministry of the dying and for the wonderful example of what a very real human being is. Your spiritual depth and your gift of humor have blessed my life.

Both Joyce Rupp and I are both grateful to the following:

✦ Hospital chaplain, Carola Broderick, who read our manuscript with the lens of her ministerial expertise and her outstanding ability to fine-tune the written word.

✦ Secretary, Linda Rudkin, whose patience grew as she tried to read the handwritten drafts and pressed on with our hasty deadlines. Her great sense of humor brought us unexpected and needed joy in our stressful moments.

✦ Editor, Bob Hamma, who blessed our manuscript with his insights and his careful attention to the details of content and style.

✦ Mark Lindahl, colleague, friend, and oncology nurse whose wisdom has graced our lives. His honest openness, and his ability to be at the bedside of the ill without bringing his own agenda has been a marvelous witness to us.

✦ To all those who have supported us and cheered us on in the making of this book, we say "thank you, thank you, thank you!"

# Imagine

BY MICHAEL PODESTA

Imagine
stepping onto a shore and finding it heaven

Imagine
taking hold of a hand and finding it God's hand

Imagine
breathing new air and finding it celestial air

Imagine
feeling invigorated and finding it immortality

Imagine
passing from storm and tempest to an
unknown calm

Imagine
waking and finding it home

When my time comes to die, I hope that Joyce Hutchison can be by my side. I have known Joyce for nearly fifteen years, first as a team member on a women's retreat and then, more recently, when I have been a hospice volunteer. She is someone I know I can trust with my life and with my death. She is truly a midwife of the dying. Her many years of experience give credence to the profound and touching way she is able to enter into the dying journey of others. Her medical expertise, her gracious spirit, and her innate wisdom have given her an approach to death that is both comforting and hope-filled. She views death as a natural part of life, seeing it as the necessary journey we all must make to reach our true home. Joyce visualizes herself as accompanying each dying person to the door that opens to the other side. She "walks them home" with loving care, quiet joy, tenderness, and compassion.

It doesn't happen much anymore in our modern era of automobiles and public transit, but in the "olden days" one would often walk a companion to his or her home. There were walks home from school, from church, from a dance, or from other social gatherings. Walking someone home allowed the opportunity to give protection and guidance to the destined dwelling place. It also provided an opportunity to reflect on life and what had just been experienced. Sometimes this walking was done mostly in silence. Sometimes there was much talking going on. In any event, the walk home was one of companionship, trust, and appreciation of each other.

So it is with Joyce Hutchison in her care and companionship of the dying. While I had heard some of Joyce's moving stories on how she has journeyed with the dying, it wasn't until I had the privilege of observing her firsthand at the bedside of patients that I learned what a gift she is to them. I learned so much from her just by watching and listening. That is how the teachings are given in this book, not by anything formal or didactic but rather, by simply getting inside the stories, being there, listening to Joyce, observing how she is present with the very ill and with their families.

Joyce was the one who first suggested that we write this book together. I readily agreed, knowing how much I had learned from being with her and believing that others could also gain insights into the process of dying through the experiences she was willing to share. I also wanted to help caregivers of the very ill, knowing how much they need support and hope. Joyce's stories tell of what it is like to die and also of how one can be with the dying. The names have been changed, but the stories are true.

The meditations and prayers I have provided with each story came after much reflection on the stories themselves and from my experience as a hospice volunteer. It is my hope that they will provide an opportunity for strength and comfort in the midst of a situation that often calls for unwavering attention and dedication.

As we were preparing the manuscript, I kept thinking of more and more people I wanted to read this book: older persons who were still in good health but would benefit from seeing how others have been given dignity and respect in their dying process, all persons who need help in understanding how to be with the dying, caregivers of the very ill so that they can be nurtured and supported in their close companionship of the dying, and chaplains, pastors, and pastoral care personnel who give so much of themselves and often need inspiration and support for their ministry.

It is with deep gratitude and much hopefulness that I offer this book to you. May we all be more aware of the blessedness of living and of dying.

—JOYCE RUPP

I have a deep love for dying patients and their families. Although I have worked in oncology and hospice nursing for over twenty years, the word "burnout" is not in my vocabulary. Being at the bedside of the dying is a life-giving experience for me.

My passion for this field of nursing developed because of the journey I walked with my husband, Gary. He was diagnosed with cancer in January of 1970 with a prognosis of six months to live. He lived twenty-four years after that with numerous treatments, hospitalizations, and crises, yet always with much hope. There were many peaks and valleys on our journey. As I sat at his bedside, nurturing and caring for him and hoping with him and our children Joe, Mike, and Julie, I was living the experience of my work firsthand. I continually prayed, especially early on, that I would know by living the experience what this was like for my patients and families. By learning this, I knew I could make a difference in the lives of others on the journey. Gary was also very committed to reaching out to those encountering a similar experience and did so at every opportunity when he was physically able.

Some of the things I learned while being with Gary have greatly influenced my care for others.

They might seem small and insignificant to an onlooker, but they can have a vital impact on the one who is involved in the process. One experience that comes to mind is when Gary was first diagnosed with cancer. We were sent by ambulance to the University of Wisconsin Hospital in Madison. Gary had just gone through major surgery prior to our going there and was trying to recuperate, as well as undergo radiation treatments to the stomach in an attempt to shrink the tumor that could not be surgically removed. The doctors told me that they didn't know how successful they would be. It was possible that he could hemorrhage again and die.

I was twenty-nine years old and Gary was thirty-four. We had three children between the ages of two and five. They were staying with Grandpa and Grandma in southern Iowa. I rented a room a few blocks from the hospital. I went there early each morning to be with Gary and I stayed as late as I could each night. I would sit beside Gary's bed while he slept or just lay quietly. He was so sick that he didn't talk much. The nurses, doctors, and certified nursing assistants would come in and out of his room and care for him. They were cordial to me and took good care of Gary.

In spite of their good care of Gary, I was filled with anxiety and fear. I was very lonesome for our children. I had never been away from them overnight. And I was scared to death about what might happen to Gary. As I sat there each day from morning until night, I yearned for one of those people who came into Gary's room to touch me. My skin felt starved for touch and I longed for a reassuring hug. Day after day I recall thinking: *I hope I can remember this when I take care of my patients and families.*

When I returned to my work as an RN, I would often recall some of the feelings that I experienced. As I cared for my patients and families, I was committed to putting myself in their shoes to the best of my ability—to strive to understand their needs. Looking back over the years, I realize that my work is a continual learning process, trying to be open, trusting the moment, and being with others in a kind and caring way.

I also learned the importance of telling the patient and family what is going on, or at least to stop long enough to inquire if they have any questions. I remember thinking that silence or no explanation meant the worst when Gary was so ill, and I found out that this wasn't always the case; sometimes it just meant that no one took the time to give explanations.

Another thing I learned was the importance of presence. Caregivers are the greatest of task-masters, busily doing all they can to help, and sometimes just stopping in to be present without a task is important. I learned about this the hard way. One Sunday after working on the oncology floor of the hospital and being extremely busy with many very sick patients, I was driving home across the freeway when I started crying. I suddenly realized that I had given every IV morphine push that was needed, completed every blood transfusion that was ordered, kept everyone's IV going, changed Hickman catheter dressings, etc.,

etc., but I hadn't looked into the eyes of a single person all through the day. I had only been attentive to physical things and had not really noticed the patients in the bed. I felt sick to my stomach and I vowed I would never do that again.

Working with dying patients is very scary for many people. Caregivers often feel inadequate and uncomfortable because the person is going to die and they can't promise them the hope that they will get better. I learned from Gary, my mom, my patients and families that dying is just a part of our journey of life. We are all on this journey and dying is a part of it for each of us. That does not mean that hope is gone. Hope just changes to a very realistic, practical hope. Hope changes from *I hope I will be cured*, to *I hope I can keep working*, to *I hope I will be able to keep eating*, to *I hope I have a comfortable death free of pain*. Sometimes hope becomes more beautiful than ever in our lives because it is about hope for the present moment and hope that is natural, such as, *I hope the sun shines today*.

This book is intended to provide caregivers and family members of the very ill a level of comfort with those who are dying and encouragement on their journey with them. I believe when we are dying is the only time in our lives when we are bare bones real people. It is the only time in our lives when there is no need for masks, no one to fool or compete with, no need for greed or jealousy, because we are dying. I feel that it is an extreme privilege for people to allow me to be a part of their life at this time on their life's journey.

Being with the dying is one of the most intimate experiences on this earth. It is very much like being in the delivery room as a baby is being born, and we all know what a miracle that is. Well, being at the other end of a person's life as he or she is preparing to be born into eternal life is as great a miracle. I often have felt that this dear, dying person that I am with is in the palm of my two hands, and I am, through my caregiving, just handing him or her back to God. I refer to caregivers of the dying as being midwives of the dying. It is the most spiritual of experiences. The love and the presence of God at the bedside as a person is taking those last few breaths is life-giving to me.

One of the greatest gifts I have received from my dying patients is a wonderful insight into what heaven, life hereafter, eternal life, or life after death might be like. I have been committed to walk beside dying persons with whatever belief systems they had, and in doing that I have been enriched spiritually by their varied beliefs. For some, their idea of heaven has been a campfire surrounded by folks who love each other, a flower-filled space with a baby, a journey with loved ones coming to meet them, or a journey of flying with the birds and feeling as free as can be. Would I have this rich view of what new life after death might be without having shared their journey? I think not. I am extremely grateful to each and every one with whom I have journeyed. They have helped me to look forward to what is waiting for me when I complete my own journey on this earth.

My husband, Gary, also helped me to see death in a life-giving way. He would listen to me as I shared my experiences about my wonderful patients and families, and he often encouraged me to write the stories down and share them with others who had similar encounters with a loved one's dying. (And so Gar, I am doing this for you. Thanks so much for inspiring me to do so.)

I hope these stories will alleviate the fears of those of you who are at the bedside of the dying. I hope they will help you to know that you can hardly go wrong if you just listen as intently as you can, be as present as possible, and above all remember that your own agenda needs to be left outside of the patient's room. This is the dying one's journey and each one does it a little differently. We need only to walk beside them with our love and support in order to be good companions for them as they journey Home.

—JOYCE HUTCHISON

## *Loved Ones*

While "loved one" is used in the prayers to refer to the one who is ill, we realize that many times we may have relational difficulties with spouses, parents, and others for whom we are caring. Some readers may not have a loving relationship with the one with whom they walk. Also, some readers may have a professional rather than a personal relationship to the one who is ill.

Therefore, we suggest that "loved one" be replaced with another word that is more fitting when the situation calls for it. "Dad, Mother, patient, sister, etc." could be substituted. Use whatever word will help the prayers to be relevant and helpful for you.

## *Caregivers*

Who are caregivers? As we wrote this book we thought of all those who accompany someone who is ill. Some central caregivers are spouses, parents, daughters, sons, and other relatives or friends who are there day in and day out. Caregivers might be living with the person who is very ill, or they may be going each day to a hospice facility, a nursing home, or a hospital to be with him or her. Caregivers are also those who supply medical help and guidance. Nurses, physicians, nurses' aides, physical therapists, and many others give constant care to the patient. There are also those significant caregivers known as chaplains, who care for the spirit of the patient with kindness and compassion.

We hope that anyone who is connected with a person who is very ill will benefit from these stories and prayers. Journeying with someone who is suffering requires much compassion, energy, and a daily restoring of faith. Caregivers need to care for themselves, and often they are so busy helping the ill one that they forget or are unable to do so. Perhaps one of these stories or prayers will bring comfort, hope, and new energy of spirit to those of you who are giving care to someone who is very ill. We know you have a tough road to walk. We understand.

## What Is Hospice?

The word "hospice" means "lodging for travelers." Those who are dying are traveling a special journey and hospice care provides these "travelers" with companionship and loving care for the final journey of life. Hospice is for anyone who has a medical diagnosis in which he or she has days, weeks, or months to live. However, the focus is not on how long someone has to live. Rather, hospice focuses on trying to help each day that a person lives be the best it can be for them, no matter how long or short their remaining time is. Hospice care strives to help the patient make good choices and to have as much control as possible in his or her medical care.

Hospice services provide for the total well-being of dying individuals and their families. This service is given by a team of trained professionals, including the patient's physician, who directs the patient's care. Hospice caregivers travel alongside the dying, offering whatever services they can provide so that the patient is able to live each day with as much comfort and peace as possible. Registered nurses help with symptom management such as relieving physical pain, nausea, breathlessness, or whatever patients might be experiencing that impedes their comfort. The nurses also teach families how to care for their loved ones and are attentive to any needs that might exist.

Social workers help patients and families cope with emotional, relational, and financial stresses. Clergy members are available to give spiritual support, if the patient desires this. Home health aides assist with personal care and help with household chores related to the patient's situation. Trained volunteers offer companionship and help with daily tasks and errands. Pharmacists, dietitians, and others with special skills are available for consultation when needed. Massage and music therapists are also often a part of the hospice team, ready to help the patient prepare for the final journey home. Grief support counselors, who provide support to family and friends after the loved one's death, are another vital part of the hospice team.

Providing comfort to patients enables them to

participate in life as fully as is possible [for them,] if they so choose. The needs of the patient and family are of vital concern to those who offer care. Hospice services are most often carried out in the home because home is where most of us want to be. If being cared for at home is not possible or preferable, however, hospice care is also available in designated hospice facilities or in nursing homes. Hospice strives to provide loving care wherever the patient's final time is spent.

Hospice caregivers have a tremendous respect and reverence for those who are approaching their death. They try never to interfere with an individual's personal beliefs and values. At the same time, hospice caregivers do all they can to assure that the physical, emotional, spiritual, and mental needs of the patient are attended so that the dying one can journey home with peace of mind and heart. As you read the following stories, you will learn from the lived experiences of the dying how to care for them as well as how to make your own journey home.

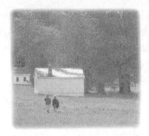

# ONE

# Giving Permission to Die

My mother was dying of cancer and I knew that she was getting close to her death. I had learned from my work with hospice that I should give her permission to die. I knew that in doing this it gave people the freedom to let go when they had been sick for so long. I had talked to families about this in the past and explained the dynamics of it, but it didn't seem to apply now. Not to my mother and me.

Mother and I had had a very meaningful relationship since her diagnosis in January. It was now the end of December and we had experienced many things. One of these was a big celebration. Her and Dad's forty-ninth wedding anniversary was in November. Since mother had talked for four or five years about having a special celebration on their fiftieth wedding anniversary, and I knew she wouldn't be with us by then, I suggested having a big celebration for their forty-ninth. I said, "If you do live until your fiftieth, we will do it again."

She was very excited and wanted the party. We had the celebration on November 29 with over two hundred people in attendance. Their marriage was blessed at a Mass that day and their six grandchildren participated in it. Mother and Dad were so proud and happy in spite of her frail little body of about ninety pounds and the oxygen concentrator sitting beside her chair at the church reception room where we had the party. It was a celebration of their marriage, but we were also aware of celebrating the gift of her life.

I had done everything I could to make this time for her the best that it could be and she was very grateful. I felt more love for her than I ever had before and I didn't want her to die. How could I tell her it was okay to die? It wasn't okay.

One evening, I was sitting beside my mother and she was sleeping. She looked so fragile and pale and her breathing was slightly labored. I knew she didn't have a long time to live. I was thinking about the fact that I hadn't been able to tell her it was okay to let go and I was feeling very burdened about this. Mother opened her eyes, smiled at me, and said, "You are such a good nurse."

I started to cry and I said, "Oh no, I'm not, Mother. You see, there is something that I know I should do for you and I haven't been able to do it. But you started this, so here I go. Mom, I know you are dying and I know *you know* you are dying. I can't stop it and you can't stop it, so as of this very moment I give you up freely and I know I will be with you again someday."

Her face filled with a radiant smile and she said, "Joyce, that is the greatest gift you have given me. I want to tell you what it is like to be dying. If you have ever left your kids with a baby-sitter and you walk away and hear them crying behind you, that is what it is like to be dying. I know I'm dying, but everyone is pulling on my shirttail to stay here. I can't stay. Your Dad is pulling the hardest. Can you talk to him?" I told her I would, but I didn't know if he would be able to let her go as he was desperate for her to live.

I did talk to Dad. I started telling him about my conversation with Mother and after only a couple of sentences, he interrupted me with, "Don't ask me to tell her it's okay to die because I am not going to do it!" I reassured him that if he couldn't, it was okay because there was no right or wrong way about doing it. I told him of the struggle that it was for me as her daughter and that I couldn't imagine what it would be like for him as her husband of forty-nine years. I also told my dad that if he didn't tell mother it was okay to die that she would understand. She knew him better than anyone else. She was very aware of the pain he felt at the thought of her leaving him.

How surprised and grateful I was when, a few hours before Mother died, Dad was actually able, through his tears, to tell Mother that it was all right to die, that he would be okay. He, too, had found the strength to let her go.

Thank you, Mom, for helping me to let go of you when the time came. Most mothers birth us and teach us how to live, but not every mother also teaches us how to die. Thank you for allowing me to accompany you as you were birthed into eternal life.

## CAREGIVER'S ✸ REFLECTION

### *Meditation*

Visualize God as a comforting mother.

Feel God's strength fill your whole being.

Imagine now that your hands are holding on tightly to your loved one.

Let God's hands enfold your hands and gently help you to open your tight grasp.

Rest in God's abiding presence as you draw strength to let go of your loved one.

### *Prayer*

Tender and consoling God,
your love is like a nurturing mother.

You know what it is like
to love with a full heart.
You understand how hard it is
for me to let go.

Assure me that the love

I have for my loved one
will live on in my heart.
My "letting go" will not diminish
our relationship.

Please help me give my loved one
permission to die.
Grant that I can find the words
to say what needs to be said.
May I have the courage to do this.

Bless our time together.

## *For Today*

I will search my heart to see if I am ready to let go
of my loved one.

If I am not ready to let go, I will pray for strength
and courage to do so.

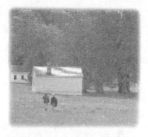

# TWO

# What's His Name?

When I first met Henry I never dreamed I'd feel so close to him when he died. He smelled of stale liquor, had a three-day stubble of gray whiskers, and had not bathed in some time. Henry was in his mid-sixties, had cancer of the lung, and lived alone in a low income apartment. He initially came to the outpatient clinic for weekly chemotherapy. I gave him many of his chemo treatments and we had lots of time to talk because each treatment took at least an hour. He told me about his life, that he was an alcoholic and hadn't been very proud of how he had lived his life. He talked about how he had basically deserted his wife and children and usually spent whatever money he made on booze. As he reviewed his life, he said he felt bad about the way he had lived it and that he had made lots of mistakes. He voiced regrets about never seeing any of his family again since he had turned his back on them because of his alcoholism.

Henry came to his oncology appointment one day having had too much to drink. That day the chest x-ray showed that the tumor in his lung was larger, which meant there was no use in continuing with chemotherapy. He was quite short of breath, very weak and frail, and was having a great deal of pain, so the doctor admitted him to the hospital. After being there a couple of days, it was obvious that Henry would never be able to go back to his apartment again. I said to the doctor one day, "We all know that Henry is getting close to dying. What if we brought some liquor to the hospital? Quality of life is important and it wouldn't be good for him to go through D.T.'s (delirium tremors) as sick and pain-filled as he is now."

The doctor agreed, and so I brought a bottle of whiskey to the hospital after work that day. I took it in to Henry and I showed him what I had. He broke into a big smile, but looked a little shocked. I said, "I brought this present to you and we will keep it at the nurses' station and you can have a drink occasionally if you want."

Henry started to open the drawer to his bedside table and was fumbling around in it, as if he were looking for something. I said, "Could I help you find something?" He said, "I want to pay you. I really appreciate this." I knew he didn't have any money, but I had also learned from all the times he shared his story with me that it was important to him that he pay his way. So I replied, "Henry, I would rather you pay me with a favor." He said, "What's that?"

I explained: "Well, you've told me that even though you've made mistakes in your life, you believe in a loving God. You believe that your God has forgiven you for your past and you feel very peaceful about where you are going when you die. Is that right?" He answered, "Oh yes, I know my God forgives me and I know I will join him when I die." So I said, "Well, I have a twin brother in heaven and I want you to tell him 'Hi' for me when you get there." Henry said, very enthusiastically, "Well, I will!"

A few days later as I was spending time with Henry, very aware of how fast he was failing, he said to me: "How do you make out a will here? I would like to make out a will." I asked the social worker to come and talk with him. After the social worker helped him make out his will, Henry shared it with me. He wanted his overcoat to go to the man down the hall in the rooming house. He wanted his shaving kit to go to another man down the hall. He wanted the canned goods in his kitchen to go to the lady who lived across the hall from him. (She used to bring him home-cooked food sometimes.) He had $15.00. He split that and wanted $5.00 to go to three friends, myself being one of them. That was Henry's will.

A few days later, the utilization review person in the hospital said Henry had to go to a nursing home because he did not require acute nursing care in a hospital anymore. Henry was very sad because the staff at the hospital had become his family. I promised him I would try to come each day to visit him if I could.

Henry was transferred to a nursing home and was there only three days before he died. I went each of those three days after work and sat with him. He could hardly speak anymore, only in a whisper, if at all. The last evening I was with him, I was just sitting quietly holding his hand, and he appeared to be unaware that I was there. He had labored breathing and was nearing death. After a while, Henry opened his eyes and looked at me for a while. His eyes were glassy and he seemed to be looking far away. Then he acted as if he wanted to say something. I got closer to him and he moved his lips. There was no sound but he mouthed: "What's his name?"

I told him his name was Joe.

Henry died that night at 1:30 a.m. I have no doubt that my twin brother got the message from me. Thank you, Henry, for allowing me to travel with you on your journey home. What a privilege to be with you.

## CAREGIVER'S ✿ REFLECTION

### *Meditation*

Sit quietly in the presence of God.

Visualize your inner self filled with God's love.

Now, think of one aspect or quality of your loved one that irritates you.

Return to the love of God within you.

Pray to accept your loved one with his (her) faults and weaknesses.

## *Prayer*

Compassionate One,
when I am irritated or discouraged
by how my loved one responds
or does not respond,
fill me with compassion and kindness.

When memories of unpleasant experiences
of the past return,
assist me in extending forgiveness.

Help me, also, to be kind to myself,
to not deny the struggles.
Soothe my sore spirit
when I find the days especially difficult.

Forgive me for my own failings
and help me to overcome any guilt I have
for not always being my best self.
You know that these days are not easy ones.

Bless both of us with your merciful kindness.

## *For Today*

I will not ignore or repress irritations and frustrations, but I will also try to be kind and considerate with my loved one when I feel this way.

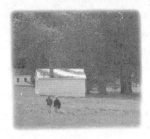

# THREE

# Why Did God Give You Cancer?

When my husband, Gary, was first diagnosed with "terminal cancer," he was thirty-four years old and I was twenty-nine. Our children were two, four, and five years of age. The doctors told Gary that he had approximately six months to live with chemotherapy and radiation. He was very sick as he went through radiation therapy, platelet transfusions, chemotherapy, and frequent hospitalizations. Two years in succession he was told that it would probably be his last Christmas.

After about four years of being in and out of the hospital many times, with countless emotional ups and downs and great uncertainty about living or dying, Gary's physical condition stabilized. He was weak, tired from the many treatments, and often "down in the dumps." It's a frustrating struggle to be told you are going to die and then continue to live, wanting to live but being a little afraid to hope that you will. At the five-year anniversary of his cancer diagnosis, Gary went back to Madison, Wisconsin, for a re-evaluation, since this was where he was told the cancer was incurable and where the treatment had been initiated. After x-rays, blood tests and scans, Gary was told there was no sign of the cancer and that it might not come back. "You mean maybe I'm cured?" Gary asked. "Yes, that's what we mean," the physicians said.

Gary and I had a lot of work to do when he came back home. You see, when we were first married, Gary was confident, social, and a very communicative person. He took care of decision-making and all of our financial matters, including paying bills. I cooked, cleaned, did laundry, and loved being a mom to our three little children. Then, when Gary got sick, I had to become stronger. I took over the responsibility of running the house and paying the bills. I had to start working full time and continue all the things I was doing before. Gary was on disability and was out of the loop of life in many ways. At the end of five years, he didn't seem to have any self-confidence, and we found that we had both changed a lot. We had almost reversed roles in our family.

Gary didn't like the person that I had become and I didn't like the person that he had become. We were each different people than we had married. Life had not been easy and yet, we both knew the commitment that we had made on our wedding day and wanted to keep it. We also were more aware than ever of what life is really about, what is important, and that the easy way is not often the right way. We knew that our love for each other was there and that what we had been through together, while being hard at times, was worth saving—even though it meant more work and effort for both of us. We sought professional help and were able to learn how to accept and love the stranger that each of us had become.

One day, Gary and I were talking about the journey we had been on—the struggles and the blessings—and I said to him, "I just don't understand why God had to give you cancer in the first place." I wondered why God was punishing us. We were trying the best we could to live right. We loved each other a lot and we loved our children. We were trying to be good parents. I repeated, "I wonder why God gave you cancer."

Gary looked at me and responded, "I can't believe you would ever believe that God gave me cancer or that he was punishing us. Joyce, that is totally wrong. Don't you believe that God is our Father? That means he is our parent—just like we are parents to Joe, Mike, and Julie. You and I both know we could not love more than we love each of our children. Even though we love them as much as we can love, they are still going to have things go wrong in their lives. They will fall or skin their knees. They could get hit by a car. They could get cancer or some life-threatening disease. Even though we love them as much as we can love, that does not prevent tough things from happening to them. Like God our Father, we can hug them, be with them in their struggle and pain, constantly reassure them, and give them strength and support. God has been doing that for us this whole time. Even though my getting cancer is part of the human condition for me, God our Father has had his arm around us all this time. He's given us love, grace, and strength to walk our journey."

This made so much sense to me. How relieved I was to hear Gary's understanding of what had happened and to be able to believe it. With his viewpoint, I could be open to God's love and not be fearful of doing something wrong. Gary gave me a wonderful gift of spiritual freedom that day and lifted a great weight from my mind and heart. He lived about nineteen years after teaching me this wonderful lesson of God's love and continued to inspire me with his peaceful faith in God.

Gary, thank you for the powerful lesson of God's love that you taught me as we journeyed together in love. The peacefulness you had as you faced your dying was the greatest of gifts for me.

## CAREGIVER'S REFLECTION

### *Meditation*

Visualize God as a kind and caring parent (a mother or a father).

Now picture yourself and your loved one who is ill.

See God coming to each of you and holding you close, as a loving parent would.

Imagine all of you in one big hug, with God's love encircling you.

## *Prayer*

Dear God,
your love is strong and enduring.
You would never deliberately harm us,
or bring us grief and heartache.
You desire only good for us.

Like a loving parent, you daily offer us
reassurance, strength, and support.

As we walk this path
filled with challenges and struggles,
your love will sustain us.

You will always be there for us.
You will forever hold us close to your heart.
Thank you for embracing us with your love.

## *For Today*

I will draw comfort from God's strong and enduring love.

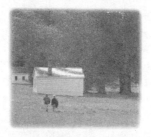

# FOUR

# A Family Journey

About 8:00 p.m., I received a call from Brenda saying, "Could you come over? It looks like my dad is taking his last breath." I left the dishes I was washing and went directly to their house, which was just a few minutes drive from my home. When I arrived, the family said Fred had started breathing again. I could tell, though, that it wasn't going to be a long time until he would die. It was then 8:10 p.m.

In Fred and Anne's bedroom, Fred lay dying. Fred was surrounded by loved ones: his wife, Anne, their two sons, Andrew and Pete, and two daughters, Brenda and Annette, along with their spouses and children. Anne sat quietly in a chair beside Fred's bed. His two adult sons lay on the bed, one on each side of their dad. Annette also sat on the bed, up by Fred's head. Two young granddaughters bounced in and out of the room, sometimes sitting on the bed for short intervals until they'd think of something they wanted to do and go into the living room to play. A college-age grandson came over to the bed and rubbed his dad's back off and on. He was quiet but very attentive to what was going on.

Everyone gave their constant attention to Fred, the dying man in the bed. Andrew reminisced about how his dad, Fred, always made them work in the garden and how, when they would get to the end of the row, they would have to quickly start on another. The other brother and sister chimed in, "But you always snuck away, Andrew, and that's why you were called 'the Shadow.'"

Brenda was the busy one, waiting on everyone, answering the phone, making coffee, doing what needed to be done. Her daughter, a grandchild of high school age, was also in and out of the room a lot. She was reflective, sad, and pensive. A very significant part of this deathbed scene was Pete's wife and their new baby, a three-week-old tiny boy, also named Fred, whom she would periodically lay in the bed beside Pete, who was lying beside his dying dad, Fred. It was an incredible scene: the beginning of life and the ending of life lying together on the same bed.

Fred's respirations were moist and rattley, sometimes very slow with long pauses between each breath. Anne and her sons and daughters urged him: "Please, dad, let go and be free." At 8:25 p.m., daughter Annette said, "Dad, you are always in bed asleep by 8:30. You better let go now and go on to heaven. You never liked to be late to bed!"

There was more reminiscing. "Dad never praised

42

us for anything," the children all agreed. "He expected a lot and it was never enough." Then Annette
recalled, "But I got a letter of apology from him once.
After he had strongly voiced his displeasure at my
decision to marry, he wrote me a letter to say he was
sorry." She said it wasn't a very long letter, only a
couple of sentences, but he did it. Anne then talked
about their dad and shared that Fred never wanted to
go to school, become a professional, or get a better
job. She said he just wanted to keep doing his regular
job of working for the post office and being at home
with her and their children. She was grateful that he
had been such a caring dad for them.

There was more labored breathing. It was now
8:45 p.m. and all of the family members were wondering if it would ever end. They told dad to quit
being stubborn and let go. Then they told him again
how much they loved him. Story after story about the
past had been shared within that slow passing hour.
As the minutes went by they listened to his every
breath, wondering if he would take another one.
Then at 8:50 p.m., Fred's breathing changed to a shallow breath and at 8:53 p.m. his breathing stopped
completely.

Even though this was the much yearned for
moment, everyone seemed shocked and sad. They
cried together, shared their relief and also their dis-
belief that he had actually died. The finality of death
is so stark and heavy. It seemed to me that something
of history and family foundation had that very second come to an end. At the same time, out of that
strong foundation, life would go on. Those whom

Fred had given life would carry that life on in their hearts and in their living.

Thank you, Fred. It was a privilege to be there as your family walked you home.

## CAREGIVER'S ✿ REFLECTION

### Meditation

Recall some of the positive qualities of your loved one.

Remember people whose lives your loved one has touched and helped.

Envision the positive qualities of your loved one's life being passed on to others.

Offer gratitude for the goodness of your loved one.

### Prayer

God of life and death,
one life ends, another begins.
The cycle occurs again and again.
Many times we do not see
this hope-filled cycle clearly
because of our pain.

What we give to others
lives on long after we die.
The goodness of a loved one

can be stored in our hearts
as an unending treasure.
This goodness can live on
into future generations.

Thank you for the hope and comfort
that this truth brings to me.
Thank you for the life and goodness
of my loved one.

## For Today

I will recognize and appreciate the good qualities of
my loved one and trust that these good qualities
will live on in the lives that he (she) has touched.

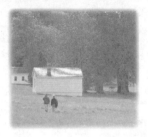

# FIVE

# Dignity and Control

It took a long time to get to know George, but it was worth it. He was a great blessing in my life. George was a farmer who was diagnosed with lung cancer several months before I met him. His family had requested help from hospice and he became my patient. I went to his home once or twice a week in the beginning to help him and his wife, Jane, with medications and to assist in getting help for his personal care. I also helped them find some volunteer assistance so Jane could get out of the house one or two afternoons a week.

George was friendly but didn't talk much about his struggle, except for his concern about what his wife was going through. I noticed several weeks after I met him that he was getting weaker and was less able to do things for himself. He could still get from the bed to the chair with help, but he couldn't walk at all. With each visit, I observed George's wife becoming more stressed and, as he grew more and more dependent, both grew increasingly discouraged.

It was clear to me that George had always taken care of everything, so this drastic change in roles was very difficult for both of them. George became quieter and more withdrawn. After doing my physical assessment and evaluating medication needs and symptom control, I would sometimes stay and sit with him without talking. He was not one to express how he was feeling. Although I cared greatly, I could do nothing to change the progression of the disease with its increasing debilitation. I knew it had to be extremely difficult for George.

One day I went to their farm and Jane said she wanted to go to the grocery store while I was there with George. He wanted to get in his chair but was extremely weak. Jane and I helped him to the chair beside his bed and then she left for the store. The nurse's aide was not scheduled until the next day so I asked George if he would like me to give him a sponge bath. He said he would like that.

During the bath George was very quiet and appeared extremely sad. He had been a large man, but was now frail and thin. He had gray, thin hair and had not shaved for a few days. After the bath, I rubbed his back, legs, and arms with lotion, shaved him, and put fresh pajamas on him. Then I fixed his recliner so he could rest. After napping for a bit, he opened his eyes and I noticed that he was staring out the picture window that was just in front of him.

After awhile I said, "You seem really down, George. Is there anything I can do?"

George continued to be very quiet for a long time and then tears filled his eyes and ran down his face. He raised his arm, pointed out the picture window, and asked: "Do you see that cornfield out there? A year ago right now I was out in that field on my tractor and now I can't even go to the bathroom without help. I'm losing it all. I've always taken care of everything, my wife and family, all the responsibilities of the farm, the bills, the finances, everything. I could keep it all going and I liked doing it. This is all so hard for my wife."

George continued to cry for a while longer. I sat silently and gently held his hand. Finally, I said, "George, I can't know what it is like for you to lose so much control over your life and to have to depend on everyone else for all that you need. It must be awful."

George started reminiscing then, about the farm and the twenty-six years they had lived there. He described the crops he had raised, told me when he bought his first new tractor, and gave me many other details of his farming life. He told numerous stories of raising his children on that farm. George became brighter and almost excited as he talked. Then he became quiet again and said somberly, "That's all gone now."

I responded, "George, as much as I want to change it for you, I can't. But, George, I do know that I am going to continue to walk beside you as much as I can for the remainder of your journey on this earth. I do know that you mean much to me, and I will be here to care for you. I will get support for your wife and be attentive to your symptoms so that you can be physically comfortable."

Again we sat quietly together. When his wife came home, she seemed refreshed and more cheerful. I prepared to leave, gathered my nurse's bag, and went to his bedside. I assured him, "George, I will be back in two days and Jane will call if you need anything before that time." I looked into his eyes and said, "I care a lot." He gave the thumbs up sign and responded, "I know you do." Our hearts touched at that moment. George lived four weeks more after that and I went to see him daily the last few days before he died.

Thank you, George, for sharing your struggle of being dependent on others and for allowing me to walk beside you on your journey. It was a privilege to be there with you.

## CAREGIVER'S ✿ REFLECTION

### *Meditation*

Sit quietly in God's presence.

Let this Loving Companion fill your mind and heart with peace.

Allow this peace to soothe you and comfort you.

See if you can entrust yourself more fully into God's care.

Now, do the same for the one you are walking home.

Entrust your loved one into God's care.

## Prayer

Jesus,
as you hung upon the cross
you knew
what it was like
to lose everything.

You knew
how painful it was
to have so little control
over your life.

Help me to be sensitive,
kind, and helpful
as my loved one
faces his (her) limitations.

May I be aware
of my loved one's struggle.
May I offer understanding
as his (her) ability to care for self
becomes less and less possible.

## For Today

I will do what I can to help my loved one have as much control over his (her) life as possible, even if it is in very small ways.

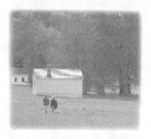

# SIX

# A Long-Kept Secret

When I was a young nurse I met a woman named Sadie who taught me so much about life, struggle, pain, and happiness. She also shared a glimpse of heaven with me. Sadie was in her early forties when we met. She was battling an aggressive breast cancer and went through many different kinds of chemotherapy and radiation. Sadie would have brief remissions, but nothing seemed to stop that cancer from raging through her body. Eventually, the breast cancer went into her bones and, consequently, she easily got fractures.

Sadie was an African American and one of the most beautiful women I have ever met, even when she lost all her hair. She had a lovely spirit and a marvelous way of welcoming everyone graciously. We spent many hours together because I was often her nurse on the oncology floor of the hospital, and I was usually the one who administered her chemotherapy treatments. I had been the nurse on duty when she was first admitted to the hospital. Sadie shared her struggles and fears with me on many occasions. She also shared the good days she had when the chemotherapy was working. She had lots of hope.

One year she was in the hospital at Christmastime. The other nurses and I had decorated her room for the holiday and it was beautiful. My children were small at the time and my husband, Gary, and I took them with us to the hospital on Christmas morning before we went out of town to visit relatives. We had a little Christmas celebration with Sadie in her hospital room. It was a special time for all of us because we knew that our coming helped Sadie to be a bit less lonely. As always, Sadie tried to be positive. Even though she was very weak and had a lot of pain with all the bone metastasis, she was cheerful and happy with my family, asking the children about their gifts and wondering how we would spend the rest of the day.

Through the next three weeks Sadie's condition deteriorated greatly. She knew she was dying, and I knew she was dying, but we didn't talk about it much. She talked to me about a lot of other things, but not about that. Sometimes we just spent quiet time together. I felt close to Sadie and loved her very much.

When I went to work one morning the staff told me that Sadie's condition had worsened during the night and she was about to die. I went to see her right after doing my reports, but she was sleeping. I was assigned to patients down the hall that day, so I wasn't able to go back into her room for several hours. I was glad she wasn't my patient that day, though, because I couldn't bear to see her dying. But in mid-afternoon I couldn't stand not to be with her. I went to Sadie's door and saw that the nurse caring for her had Sadie turned on her side with her back toward the door.

Her body was so still, I thought maybe Sadie was sleeping again. I quietly walked into her room so that I wouldn't awaken her. When I got about halfway across the room she said with a weak voice, "Joyce?" I whispered, "Yes, it's me." Sadie said, "I could tell it was you by your footsteps." Then she said, "I've been waiting for you to come in. I have something to tell you." I pulled up a chair to the side of the bed and she said, "You know I've told you almost everything about me except one thing, and I want to tell you that now."

Sadie spoke softly, revealing her secret: "When I was a very young girl I had a baby and she died at birth. I haven't told people about my baby because I was a teenager and unmarried." She went on to say: "I have often thought about my baby and felt deep sadness. Well, last night I dreamed I was in a room full of flowers and I was holding my baby. She was beautiful and I can't wait to see her when I die. I know now that I'm ready to go."

Both of us cried after Sadie had released her secret to me. They were tears of relief for her finding inner freedom and peace. They were also tears of gratitude because she had trusted me enough to risk sharing this great secret that she had kept hidden in her memory for so long.

I thanked her for trusting me with what she needed to say. Then we were quiet together while we each treasured what had just happened. Sadie died later that night.

Thank you, Sadie, for giving your secret to me so that you could go in peace. Thank you for allowing me to accompany you on your journey home.

## CAREGIVER'S ❖ REFLECTION

### Meditation

Imagine that God has a secret for you.

Hear God whisper this secret in your ear:

"I am with you. I will be your strength.

I will draw you close to my heart."

Imagine God whispering this secret to your loved one too.

### Prayer

God of far-seeing eyes,
you know what is deep within us;
you love us as we are.

Help my loved one
to release
anything that keeps him (her)
from being free.

May I be a good companion
for the birth of this freedom
by my openness
and my non-judgment.

And God,
teach us the secrets
of your heart,
for they are the truths
of your great kindness
and compassion.

## For Today

I will listen and be open to whatever my loved one
wants to share with me.

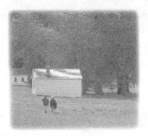

# SEVEN

# The Gift of Humor

I once cared for an older man who was of meager means and facing the end of his life. Cecil was diagnosed with lung cancer some months before I met him and his body was already beginning to show signs of deterioration. He was about 5'6" tall and weighed around eighty-five or ninety pounds. His eyes looked tired much of the time and his face was always a pasty white. Cecil was still able to manage by himself in the apartment where he lived, but movement was painful for him. He moved slowly and was slightly bent over when he walked.

On my visits to his home, we would spend part of our time talking about symptoms he was having and what medications needed to be adjusted to help him be comfortable. Then we would spend time talking and listening to one another. Cecil shared his life story with me. He loved to fish, so he told me lots of fishing stories. I could tell that he had enjoyed life.

Although I spoke about some of my life with him, I mostly listened. His stories and his love of life nestled deep in my heart.

I went back as often as Cecil needed either medication or other support to cope with his illness, so I saw him quite frequently. He gradually got weaker and it was difficult for him to care for himself. It was then that his ninety-two-year-old mother, Grace, moved in with Cecil to help with his care. She was every bit as delightful and gracious as he was. Cecil's mother was a tiny little woman with long white hair wrapped up in a small knot on the back of her head. She was extremely frail in appearance, but the peaceful strength in her nurturing, care-giving, and loving of her son will always be with me. I could tell her heart hurt to watch her own son journey toward his death, and yet she never hesitated a second in her constant presence and love of him. Like Cecil, she had nothing of material means, but I often thought "I want to be like Grace when I grow up."

They shared many stories in my presence—stories of his growing up years, of his two sisters and him playing together, of mom's cooking and baking cookies for them, of picnics with the whole family when the ants seemed to eat as much as they did. The love these two shared was readily apparent in their stories and in the easy way they related to one another.

I continued to monitor Cecil's level of comfort and to help his mother understand why he couldn't eat and that it was all right if he didn't. At that stage of his illness, food would not have made a difference. This was very difficult for Cecil's mom. One of the powerful ways that she had shown her love for him all of his life was to cook for him and make good things for him to eat. I encouraged her to do other nurturing things for him like rub his skin with lotion and put cool washcloths on his forehead.

Cecil talked to me about his dying and he began welcoming it more and more. He was sure that there was fishing in heaven and seemed sometimes to be more focused on life beyond death than on the present moment. I loved being with him and his mother even though they were sad and I was sad for them. We were on the journey together and there was a certain comfort in this. Cecil's frail little mother never stopped being a mother with her nurturing and her unconditional love. These two people never had much in material things, but they had something deeper that sustained them.

One day, toward the end of his life, I was sitting with Cecil. He was very weak and didn't talk much anymore. He looked at me and whispered, "It's getting close." I held his hand and said, "I love you and I'm going to miss you." He was quiet for a moment and then assured me, "We will be together again someday." I smiled at him and quipped, "I hope I make it!" He got a sparkle in his eye and remarked, "Well, if you get close, I'll throw you a rope." We laughed together—right there in the midst of his dying. It was a precious moment when our two hearts touched.

Thank you, Cecil, for assuring me that you would be there when I end my journey and for allowing me to walk with you as you completed yours.

# CAREGIVER'S � REFLECTION

## *Meditation*

Close your eyes and picture God's being there with you and your loved one.

See a look of love on God's face.

Let yourself feel the joy that God has for you and your loved one.

## *Prayer*

Joy-filled Presence,
there are many days
when the last thing I want to do
is smile or have a good laugh.
This caring for a dying one
is tough.
It takes its toll on the human spirit.

Help me to find moments
in the day
when I can smile.

Help my loved one and me
to laugh together,
to find the little joys of life
that sustain and uplift us.

Remind us often
that you are with us.

I'll let my eyes smile even if my face can't. I'll listen closely to see if there are a few things we can enjoy together even if it is a difficult day. I'll try not to feel guilty if I laugh with visitors. And I'll remember that you are with each of us, God.

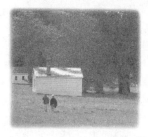

# EIGHT

# Close Enough to Touch

Viola was a dynamic, intelligent woman whom I met some years ago while I was working in oncology. She had been diagnosed with colon cancer and because she was a woman who had always taken charge of her life, she did much study and research about colon cancer and the various treatments available to her. She had many questions for the oncologist and would sometimes have to take a few days to contemplate her decisions about the treatment that was suggested for her. She was never rude or demanding in her need to have questions answered but was very deliberate and thorough in discussing the research that she had done.

When I first met Viola, I sometimes felt intimidated because she always had so many questions and did her homework so thoroughly. I feared that I might not know the answers to her questions about the chemotherapy treatments that I was administering to her. She was so articulate and confident in her communication that she scared me.

The possibility of there not being a cure for Viola's cancer was simply not an option for her. She didn't want the doctor or anyone to give up hope because, after all, "research is constantly being done so maybe something new will be discovered tomorrow that will bring a cure for me."

Five days out of each month she came to the oncology office where I gave her the prescribed chemotherapy. It wasn't long until we developed a friendship and my fears and intimidation were gone. We had time those five days each month to do a lot of talking. Viola would describe her fears, her dreams, her life. I enjoyed being with her as she was very insightful and reflective. Each month she would share more of herself with me and I with her.

We were side by side on her journey of living with the colon cancer that had metastasized to the liver. The chemotherapy held it in check for several months and then she became quite ill. Viola was admitted to the hospital for tests and intravenous feeding because she had been vomiting and was dehydrated. Each morning, at the end of our daily rounds, I went to see her for awhile. One morning I walked into her room and sat down beside her and asked her how it was going. She told me she knew things were worse, but all the scans weren't completed yet so she didn't know how extensive the cancer had become.

Viola told me she was discouraged. We were

quiet for awhile. Then, I expressed my concern for her and she said to me, "You always touch me or hold my hand when you are with me." I told her that I didn't realize I had done that and I hoped I had not offended her.

She responded, "Not at all. It means a lot to me. You see, most people come to my door or my bedside and they remain a distance away as they ask me how I am. I know if I share my struggles that they will be gone in a flash because they are so uncomfortable and seem afraid of what I might say. It seems by their distance that they are going to make a quick exit if I talk about anything very serious. But you, you come in and you sit down, if only for a little while, and you take my hand or lay your hand on my arm. It seems like you have made a commitment to me by doing that. I know that no matter what I say or how much I talk about my fears, my dying, or my sadness, you are going to be with me for however many minutes I share my struggle with you. You won't leave me or act like what I'm saying is too much for you. When you touch me, I feel like you commit yourself to listening to me in the moments ahead."

Viola said that touching shows commitment. Wow! She taught me volumes by her words and I would not have known it if we had not risked sharing on a deeper level. By being very present to her and walking beside her on her journey to death, Viola taught me how to be with others who are facing their dying.

Thank you, Viola, for our time together. You touched my life as I walked you home.

## *Meditation*

Visualize Jesus as he was with the sick and the dying.

See how he places his hands on many of them.

Notice how loving he is.

Now close your eyes and see Jesus place his hands gently upon you as a blessing.

Then see him do the same with your loved one.

## *Prayer*

God who reaches out
and touches,
help me to experience
your embrace today.
Come and touch
my loved one
who is dying.

May the touch
of your courage
give us what we need
during this time
of letting go.

May the touch
of your love
comfort us
and bring us
your peace.

## For Today

I will be aware today of touching the one whom I am walking home. Each time I do so, I know that God will also be touching my loved one with care and compassion.

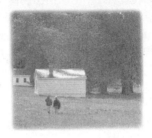

# NINE

# Always a Bit of Hope

Hope is something that people might think of as impossible for someone who is dying. Yet, patients who are dying have demonstrated that it is possible to hope for certain things in this life even when they are aware that they are near death. There was a man with whom I journeyed many years ago who taught me about having hope even as he faced the nearness of his last days.

When I first met John he had just been diagnosed with lung cancer and was starting chemotherapy and radiation treatments. He was married and he and his wife, Corinne, had a good relationship. They obviously loved each other a lot and had fun together. He had recently retired and she was still working as a secretary. They joked about how he had become "the chief cook and bottle washer" and had dinner ready every evening when Corinne got home. He teased her by saying, "The wages aren't all that great but I sure have a happy, more rested wife since I've become her maid."

John shared a lot about his life as I administered his chemotherapy to him. He was very hopeful that he would be cured of his disease. He talked about how much he regretted the fact that he had smoked for so many years, and even though he had quit smoking four years earlier, he supposed it wasn't soon enough. Still, he felt confident that he might make it through the lung cancer and have many years to live.

Eight months later a chest x-ray revealed that the tumor in John's lung was growing. The present chemotherapy was no longer helpful and every other kind of chemotherapy that was effective for that type of lung cancer had already been tried with John. After talking to his doctor, John and his wife decided that they would not try any other medical procedures. They decided that they would go home and that Corinne would care for John there.

There was no hospice in the city at that time, so another RN and I visited them regularly to help monitor John's care. Every time I went to John's home, he would tell me more about himself. On one visit, John was sitting in his recliner chair in the living room and he said to me: "I love my chair. I hope I will always be able to come out here and sit in my chair." On another visit he told me that he hoped that he could stay home and not go to the hospital again. We reassured him that, if at all possible, we would help him to stay at home. At another time John said to me,

"My grandchildren are going to visit us on Sunday. I hope they can come often. I love to see my grand-children." He was continuing to hope even during that late stage in his illness.

When I went to visit on the day before John died he was extremely weak but very alert. He slept during much of my visit, but did manage to talk a little bit. It was a rainy day. At one point he turned to me and said, "I hope that the sun shines tomorrow."

As I left John that day, I held the word "hope" in my heart. I thought about how hope sometimes changes from day to day for a dying person but that there can always be a piece of hope in their lives. As I looked back on my time with John, I saw how each one us who took care of him tried to nurture his hopes. We tried to affirm something each day that he could look forward to. We tried to be excited or happy with him, knowing these hopes brought him joy. We did this by simply being in those moments with him, allowing him to be hopeful as he moved nearer to his death.

I am grateful for this gentle, hope-filled man. He had an inner peace that radiated in his daily outlook on life. As I listened to his hopes change from the big hope of desiring a cure, to hoping for tomorrow to come, to simply hoping for today, John helped me see how even the littlest of hopes can bring a bit of joy into a dark day.

Thank you, John, for showing me that hope has many sizes and that it can help us have joy and peace as we journey home.

# CAREGIVER'S ✾ REFLECTION

## Meditation

Imagine God coming, holding out a bouquet of flowers to you.

God speaks to you: "Enjoy the beauty of these gifts today. They are yours."

Receive the flowers from God. Let your heart find hope.

Talk to God about your hope, or your lack of it.

## Prayer

God of hope,
you never stop believing in us.
You are always present with us,
assuring us that you care for us,
encouraging us to not lose hope.

Help me to find little glimmers of hope
in even the worst of days.

Inspire me to find something to believe in
when it seems there is nothing left
for me to hold on to.

Help my loved one to find something
to look forward to each day.
Together let us not lose heart.

## For Today

I will try to find a piece of hope for my loved one and for myself, just for today.

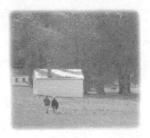

# TEN

# Will I Be Significant?

When my husband, Gary, was diagnosed with cancer and was told that he had six months or less to live, one of the hardest things for me was that I couldn't change the situation. As a wife and mom, I seemed to most always be able to make things okay for Gary and my children, but in this situation, I felt helpless. I couldn't take Gary's sadness and struggle away. I couldn't protect the kids from the fact that their dad was probably going to die. I felt helpless much of the time.

Our three active, healthy children were the positive force in our lives when everything seemed discouraging. They were a good distraction for us. My goal was to have Gary be as happy as possible at all times because he was going to die. I didn't concern myself with my own happiness. I thought: "I have many years to live. I can be happy later on." I didn't have a lot of companionship from him as he slept a lot and was often irritable or withdrawn when awake. When I would inquire about what was going on with him, he would say, "I'm just tired," or "I don't feel good."

I decided we needed a few days away to relax and enjoy being alone. We looked forward to our trip and were able to get all the arrangements made for child care—a major production as the children were now four, six, and seven. Finally, we had time away to take walks, listen to music, go to movies, shop, take naps, and just talk without interruption. Gary didn't always feel well, but we were elated just being together.

Gary talked a lot about what it was like to be dying and said it was still very hard for him to believe that he was going to die as soon as the doctor had predicted. He said losing his job was more painful than having cancer because he felt rejected, like a failure. Gary told me that having the cancer was not his fault, but somehow losing his job felt like his fault. I listened and reassured him as much as I could. I often told him of my love for him and that I would do everything to keep the house running smoothly. We talked about continuing to be honest with the kids about what was going on. We were often sad when sharing our concerns or feelings, but we also drew strength from one another when we talked honestly with each other.

One evening Gary seemed more quiet and discouraged than usual. When I asked what was going on he finally disclosed, through his tears, that he had been thinking a lot about what life would be like here when he was gone. The hardest thing for him to face about dying was the thought that when he died, he would soon be forgotten. He said he knew the kids and I loved him very much but that when he died it would be like "a grain of sand on a beach." Gary said, "Life will just go on, as it should, and everyone will soon go on with their lives and another grain of sand will fall in my place."

Gary had told me many times that he wanted me to share my life with someone else when he died. He repeated this desire of his. He continued talking, explaining how he realized that we can love people very much and yet, when they die, life goes on for the ones remaining. Other people and events start to fill the lives of those left behind. It was hard for him to face his feeling of insignificance, thinking that we would forget him when he was gone. I knew that Gary was grieving the loss of his human presence on earth.

No matter how much I tried to reassure him that he would always be present to us in our hearts, he remained sad. I felt sad for him. I hurt with him. I could not change the fact that he was sad about thinking of leaving us. I did, however, continually remind him of our love for him. The time we had being honest and open with each other and the ongoing dialogue after that trip, as he processed his grieving the loss of himself, enriched our love for each other. We knew that we were on the journey together and that was what counted the most.

Thank you, Gary, for the great significance that you have had in my life and for sharing your journey with me. I love you.

# CAREGIVER'S ✿ REFLECTION

## *Meditation*

Recall the verse of Isaiah 43:4 in which God speaks to the soul:

"You are precious in my eyes . . . and I love you."

Hear God speak these words to you.

Imagine God holding your loved one close

and whispering these words into your loved one's ear.

## *Prayer*

Loving Creator,
you have formed us
and given us
our human lives.

We are always significant
in your eyes.
You will forever love us
and never forget us.

When my loved one
raises questions
grant me an attentive,
listening spirit.

Help me to assure
my loved one

that there will always be
a place of love
in my heart for him (her).

## For Today

I will find a way in words or actions to assure my
loved one that I will always treasure his (her) place
in my life.

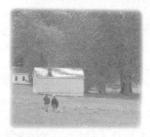

# ELEVEN

# My Last Christmas

I met Rose when I was giving her chemotherapy for breast cancer. She was a pretty, brown-eyed woman with red hair and a fair complexion. She was small in stature, well-dressed, and had a great deal of class. Rose had been diagnosed soon after the birth of her third child, a little girl. She was heartbroken with the diagnosis and each time she came for chemotherapy, she would talk to me about her fears of not being cured of cancer. She agonized over the thought of dying and leaving three children, especially her little girl, not yet two years old. Rose knew she had a very aggressive cancer and that her chances of a cure were extremely slim. Several months after we met, she developed bone metastasis and, at that point, she knew she would probably die of the breast cancer.

Rose and I became quite close because I spent much time with her giving bimonthly chemotherapy treatments. She talked to me about her family, her husband, parents, siblings, and children. She was a very loving person—kind, sensitive, and brave. Rose told me about her fears, about how she was a worrier and a perfectionist. She also shared her joys, especially how much she loved being a wife and mother.

She would sometimes apologize to me about talking so much about herself and her struggles. I told Rose that I didn't mind at all and if she ever needed to talk when she was at home, she could call. She said that the nights were the worst because that was when she would become scared and feel all alone. In the darkness of the night when everyone was sleeping, she would think of all that was ahead of her. She especially searched for reasons for why she had to die when she had three small children.

One night at 3:30 a.m., my phone rang. As I answered, I heard a little voice say, "You said I could call anytime." It was Rose and she explained that she had been awake for a long time and for some reason she just kept thinking about next Christmas (several months away). She said, "I know I won't be here and I can't imagine Christmas happening in my family without me. Who will put up the Christmas tree and do the shopping?" She continued, "It feels awful to me to think that someone else will be doing the shopping for the children. I feel sad that my husband will have to do it all alone. I sit here looking at everything in my house and how I have decorated it the way I want. Soon I will not be here. I guess it really doesn't matter anymore about how my house is decorated. . . . And how will the kids do without me? Tammy won't even remember me. . . . And how

will Katie be a teenager without me to help her. . . ?
And Matt is his mama's boy. . . . How will he ever
understand my not being here?"

Rose cried and cried as she talked on and on
about everything that was troubling her. I had no
solutions or answers for her, only a listening ear and
a deep compassion for her. I told her that I couldn't
totally understand what it must be like for her, but I
assured her that I would continue to walk beside her
and be with her on her journey. She talked to me until
6:00 a.m. when my alarm rang. I told Rose that I had
to get ready for work.

She seemed more peaceful and said that she
thought she could sleep again as she was tired and it
was finally daylight. She said her husband would get
up with the children. One last thing she added was, "I
can't imagine how Jason can get along without me as
we love each other so much and I have to leave him."
I cried with her when she said this. Then she hung up
and went to bed and I got up and went to work.

We had many other times together as she
processed letting go and talked about her dying.
Rose was very courageous as she prepared her family to be without her. She talked at great length to
Jason about leaving him and what life might be like
for him. She gave him suggestions about how to help
the children deal with her death.

Rose, you gave so much of yourself to Jason and
your three children. Your spirit lives on in their lives.
Thank you for the extreme privilege to allowing me
to walk beside you through your dark night on your
journey home.

## *Meditation*

Sit with your hands on your lap. Open your hands, palms up.

Place all your fears, worries, and concerns in your hands.

Give these all to God.

Now, place your loved one in your open hands.

Entrust your loved one into God's loving care.

## *Prayer*

Spirit of Peace,
you know how worry and fear
can take over and hound
a person's tranquillity.

Today I place my loved one,
with all his (her) worries and fears,
in your caring hands.
I place myself and my concerns
in your caring hands, as well.

Calm our hearts and minds.
Encourage us to face what troubles us.
Help us each to let go of what we fear.

Breathe your peace
through our anxious hearts,
and deepen our trust
in your abiding presence.

## For Today

I will be attentive to any worries or concerns about the future that my loved one has. I will offer assurance of my love. I will also be attentive to my own worries and concerns and try to entrust them into God's loving care.

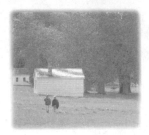

# TWELVE

# The Gate Won't Open

Bill was an elderly man who came to the hospice facility from the hospital. He was very ill but alert and talkative. He loved to visit with the staff. Bill was unable to do any of his own self-care, and one of the things that the nurse and an aide would do for him was to put him in the whirlpool bathtub when he wanted. When Bill was in there, he would talk and talk to them about his life. He shared some fairly "spicy" stories of his past and things he had done.

Bill had a twinkle in his eye, a sense of humor, and prided himself in being "a ladies' man." He was a rugged looking guy, a big built man in the past, but now, with only limited activity for so long, his flesh hung from his large frame. He would sometimes make rather filthy remarks to his women caregivers, and we would have to set boundaries for him.

Sometimes he would get irritable and gruff and snap at the staff. At first, it seemed that he was hardened through and through, but it soon became clear that he was a marshmallow on the inside. He was a lonely man who just wanted to have people in his life who cared about him.

Bill's pain was well controlled with medication, but he was getting weaker all the time. His wife came to visit almost every day, but usually she stayed only a short time because they didn't get along very well. They were distant and detached from each other and her coming seemed mostly out of duty.

As Bill's condition worsened and his dying became more imminent, he became extremely restless. He was bed-bound by now and medication didn't help him very much. Kimberly, the nurse's aide who was caring for him, came to me and asked me if I would come and see Bill because he was very agitated and seemed scared. She had bathed and shaved him, given him oral care, put clean linens on his bed and a fresh gown on him, and then given him his pain medication. In spite of all this care, she was sure that something was bothering him, perhaps something beyond his physical needs.

I went in to spend some time with Bill. I sat down and put my hands on his shoulder and arm. He had not spoken much for a few days and he didn't appear to be alert. I wasn't sure if he was able to be aware of my presence, but after sitting with him for a while I tried to communicate with him. I said, "What is the matter, Bill? Can you tell me what is bothering you?"

After a time, he said, "They won't open the gate."

He became even more agitated, repeating loudly, "They won't open the gate," as he tossed around and struggled to move. I sat thinking about that for a while, wondering what it might mean. Then a thought came to me. I told Bill that I would like to have him listen to me if he could because there was something I wanted to tell him.

I held his hand and stroked his brow to assure him of my loving presence. I talked softly into his ear and said, "Bill, it is not time for the gate to open. It will open when it's time, but for now you need to be here with us. Just let us love you and care for you. Then, when this journey is done, the gate will open and your God will be there for you."

Tears ran down Bill's cheeks. I continued, "Just be calm. There is nothing you need to do. A place is already being prepared for you and the gate will open when it is time." Bill relaxed, became calm, and I sat quietly with him. After awhile I repeated, "Just be present to this moment, Bill. We are going to be with you on your journey and we will walk you there. We will not leave you. Then the gate will open when it is time. It isn't time yet." He became very calm, dropped off to sleep, and died a few days later. After our time together Bill was not restless or fearful again.

Bill, thank you for sharing your fears with me and for allowing me to accompany you to that open gate that led you home.

## *Meditation*

Picture God waiting for your loved one by the gate of Eternal Life.

See how God opens the gate and welcomes him (her).

Notice what a blessed reunion this moment is.

Let yourself feel the happiness of this welcome.

## *Prayer*

Divine Gate-Keeper,
you alone know the time
when my loved one will depart
from this side of life.

You wait at the gate
of eternal life,
assuring each one of us
that there is nothing to fear.
Your everlasting kindness
fills the open gate
and promises us peace.

We cannot hurry the journey
and we cannot stop the journey.

Grant patience and trust to both of us
as we await the moment

when the gate will open,
and your presence will welcome
my loved one home.

May peace fill our minds and hearts.

## *For Today*

I will try to be patient with the dying process of my loved one. I will extend this patience to all who are involved in his (her) care.

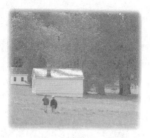

# THIRTEEN

# How Do I Do It?

I met this lovely woman and her daughter on a sunny day in June. She lived in a small town in a pretty little house with flowers all around it. There was a tiny greenhouse in the back yard with birdhouses and bird feeders hanging around it. The first day I went to see Anna I noticed how beautiful the flowers were. I entered the back door of her little bungalow and walked into the kitchen where I found her sitting in a rocking chair. Her daughter was there and graciously welcomed me.

Anna had been diagnosed with cancer of the gallbladder a couple of years before and had undergone chemotherapy. She said the chemo made her very sick, and she had to be in the hospital because her blood counts were so low. The cancer had spread and she was tired of going through treatments. She just wanted to stay home and let "nature take its course."

Anna loved her flowers, her yard, and her home, and she wanted to stay there for the remainder of her life. Her daughter was supportive of her mother's wishes and assured her that she would stay with her when Anna was no longer able to be alone.

Anna had a turban on her head the first few times I went to see her. Eventually, she seemed more comfortable just letting me be with her, with the very small amount of short fine hair covering her head. Each time I went to her home she seemed more relaxed. Eventually, I wasn't company anymore, just one of the few folks who was walking the final journey with her.

She became weaker quite rapidly and agreed to have a hospital bed brought into her home. Although Anna struggled with giving up her own bed, she knew she needed to be able to raise the head of the bed for better breathing. She had had no pain up to this time but then developed severe abdominal pain, requiring morphine to control it. She was a very stoic woman and I believe she had pain much longer than she admitted because she was used to enduring difficulties in her life.

Her daughter, Jenny, stayed in her home full time after that and had a loving, caring relationship with her mother. Anna often voiced her great appreciation for Jenny's attentiveness. Though she had five other children, Jenny, her youngest, had been her helper and companion after Anna's husband had died several years earlier. Anna continued to talk about her little house and hoped she would have more time in it to enjoy her flowers and the birds, but once she realized that she was rapidly getting weaker, she expressed a desire to die and wished she wouldn't linger a long time.

I went to see her on Friday and told Jenny that her mother probably had only a few days to live. Anna was alert but drowsy and talked about being glad she was in her home rather than the hospital. She didn't want to take too much pain medication. She voiced her need to be alert and in charge of what was happening as much as possible. When I inquired about any fears she might have, Anna said she wasn't afraid and felt everything was going well, again voicing her gratitude that Jenny was there.

Jenny and I talked several times on the weekend. I answered her questions and offered her reassurance as she watched her mother's journey getting shorter. Early on Monday morning I drove to their home and could tell that Anna was dying. She was alert and told me she was ready to go. She then asked me what she needed to do to die. I reassured her that she didn't need to do anything. She had nothing to do but just wait until it was time. We talked about the birds outside her window, and I suggested that when it was time she could fly away with her dear birds. She seemed to relax more when I told her there was nothing for her to do. She had been so used to taking care of everything or doing what needed to be done that she was sure she needed to do something in order to die.

Her daughter and son-in-law, Chuck, told her it was okay to let go when it was time to fly away. They would be all right, so would the rest of the family. It was about thirty to forty-five minutes more before she died. Anna would sleep and then awaken slightly. She seemed peaceful and relaxed. Then her breathing changed and within a few minutes Anna didn't breathe again.

What a beautiful woman you were, Anna—a woman of nature, a woman who lived a simple yet a very rich life. Thank you, Anna, for sharing your final journey among the flowers with me. It did seem as though you flew away with the birds as you made your way home.

## CAREGIVER'S 🕸 REFLECTION

### Meditation

Imagine God holding out a basket to you.

Place your questions, doubts, and concerns in the basket.

Let God take care of the basket for you.

### Prayer

Abiding Presence,
you are waiting for my loved one
to come home to you.

You will show him (her) the way.
Help my loved one to wait confidently.

Teach us both how to let go
when the time comes.
Help him (her) to be comfortable
in "doing nothing" as he (she) prepares for death.

Guide and direct us as we experience
the mystery of dying.

Thank you for being with us.

## *For Today*

My open hands will remind me that I have placed
all in God's care.

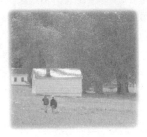

# FOURTEEN

# I'm So Ready to Go

Maurice was one of the most handsome men I have cared for in hospice. His thick black hair was just beginning to gray and he had deep brown-black eyes and dark olive skin. Maurice had inner beauty as well. I first met him when I went to care for him in the hospice room at the nursing home. He had just moved there from his own home. He was living with cancer of the lung and he became weaker and unable to care for himself. Maurice had fallen a few days earlier at home and that was his sign that he couldn't be alone any longer. His son came from Oregon to help him make arrangements to leave his home and move to the care center.

When I visited with Maurice, he would have to rest after every few sentences because he was so short of breath. He talked about his frustration with his new environment, how it was so different from home: people in other rooms yelling, having food brought to him on schedule whether he felt it was time to eat or not, and being awakened to take medicine. The room felt foreign and unwelcoming to him. Each time I went to visit him, Maurice was weaker, but he still was able to tell me more and more about himself and his life.

His favorite subject was his wife, Vivian, who had died three years earlier on Memorial Day. Each time I came he talked at great length about how much he loved her, what good friends they were, how he met her, and the fun things they did together. Maurice talked about the difficult adjustment he and Vivian had with their move to a small town in Iowa. He had been a career man in the service and they had lived in many different places. After his retirement from the army he and his wife had traveled and explored areas of interest in the U.S., as well as overseas. They both shared an enthusiasm about history and enjoyed learning through their travels. They chose a small town in which to retire because Vivian had grown up there and thought it would be a good place to live out their old age.

It was such a different lifestyle than they were used to, but they were both pretty open and flexible and it had gradually become home to them. They had formed good friendships and he joked about the fact that they both seldom met a stranger where they lived.

One day he told me about their last trip just before she died. He said Vivian had a "bad heart" and had been going to the doctor for it. One day she told Maurice that she wanted to take the Amtrak train to Oregon to visit their two sons when she was feeling stronger. Maurice said, "I was determined to take her there, although I was scared about going because I didn't know if she was well enough." He confided that the most favorite thing in the world for him was making her happy because she had brought so much happiness to him.

They did make the trip to Oregon and she tolerated the travel quite well. They had been at their son's only a few days, though, when she suddenly became very ill in the morning. She and Maurice were there alone because his son was at work, so Maurice called an ambulance. They made it to the hospital, but Vivian died that same day. Maurice told me that his wife was the most important person in the world to him and that he was ready to go and be with her. He talked about the fact that she was his world and that there just wasn't life without her.

The next time I went to see Maurice he was much weaker and had more labored breathing. He appeared to be failing fast and I knew he would be dying soon. I talked with him about his condition and about the fact that he was dying. He responded by telling me that it was hard to try to make himself get better. He seemed to have lost his desire to live. Maurice said again that he was quite ready to die and had no fear of dying, in fact he said he looked forward to it. He talked some more about his life, telling me that he had had a good life and it would soon be time to go. He was increasingly short of breath and it became more difficult for him to talk.

I sat with him for thirty minutes while he slept. He awakened and again spoke of his wife and of his excitement to see her when he died. I reassured him that we would see that he had the medication he needed to be comfortable. In case I did not see him again before he died, I thanked him for sharing his life with me. This was Friday. On Sunday evening, Maurice died very peacefully.

Thank you, Maurice, for sharing the story of your love for your wife and for your joyful anticipation of journeying home to her.

## CAREGIVER'S 🕸 REFLECTION

### Meditation

Rest quietly. Be assured that you are not alone.

God is with you.

Remember deceased people whom your loved one especially appreciated.

Picture these special persons welcoming your loved one as he (she) dies.

Imagine the joy and love that they extend to your loved one.

### Prayer

Welcoming God,
you are ready to receive my loved one
when he (she) departs from this life.

May this waiting welcome
be a source of courage for my loved one
as he (she) dies.

Constantly remind both of us
that dying is not an ending,
but rather, a beginning of new life.

May the friends and relatives who have died
be there to greet my loved one.

May his (her) passing-over be gentle
and the final journey be peaceful.

## *For Today*

I will remember that my loved one is making a journey to a new home.

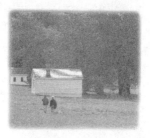

# FIFTEEN

# A Friend Dies

Stephanie was in her early twenties when we met at a church retreat. She was a lovely young woman, and even though I was forty-five we seemed to bond that weekend. Stephanie shared her deep desire to meet a nice man, marry, and have children. I told her I would add her to my prayer list, as I highly recommended marriage and family. She was also a nurse and had just started working on the oncology floor of the hospital, so we had much in common.

Through the next several years our paths crossed, sometimes frequently and sometimes only occasionally. She did marry a man from her hometown and gave birth to two little girls who were her life. She continued in nursing as a part-time hospice nurse and then she started working with cancer research doing studies with oncologists. Since I worked in an oncology office, we saw each other more often then and enjoyed our frequent, brief chats. We truly were special friends.

I then left oncology to work full-time with hospice. Several months after leaving the oncology office, I discovered that Stephanie had cancer. What a shock. When I went to see her she told me her story. She had sinus trouble and had been seeing the doctor for it for several weeks when the physician became suspicious. Stephanie was taken to surgery and they found cancer of the sinus. She was undergoing radiation therapy and was hopeful that maybe they could cure the cancer.

I continued to keep in touch with Stephanie, and she was quite well for almost a year. Then she had a recurrence. She underwent more radiation treatments, but she knew her prognosis was poor. Stephanie's hope was shattered. Her little girls were five and two at the time.

One day I had just come into the hospice office after seeing my patients and sat down at my desk to chart. My phone rang and a voice said, "Joyce, this is Stephanie and I have a favor to ask. I'm ready for hospice and I would like you to be my hospice nurse." Even though I knew what her prognosis had been, I was shocked. "Of course," I said, "I would be privileged to be your nurse." I went to Stephanie's home the next day and admitted her to hospice. I listened to her hopes, her plans, her fears, and her frustrations.

Because Stephanie was a nurse, she directed her self-care as much as she chose. Her husband was scared and helpless. Stephanie had definitely been the caretaker and director in the family. She wanted to do everything that she could to help Mike and the girls cope when she was gone. We assisted her in making movies for them to have, in writing letters, and even helped her make a ceramic hand print of herself for each one of the girls so when they got lonesome they could put their hand in hers. She became weaker each day and had to increase the dose of pain medication often to keep up with the intense pain.

I went to see Stephanie on Tuesday morning, even though I had just been there the day before, because I knew her condition was deteriorating quickly. It appeared that she was dying, so I called Mike to come home from work and her mom to come from her home, which was an hour away. Stephanie was lucid at times but only semi-responsive much of the time. I didn't leave her house that day as she needed frequent medication and dose monitoring. I assured her that I would be with her.

Stephanie's every waking moment was spent with concern for her two little girls, her husband, her mom—everyone but herself. The girls played about the house and sat on her bed. They cried sometimes because Mommy didn't respond like she always did. We reassured them and answered their questions appropriately. Stephanie died very slowly, it seemed by inches, as we all sat around her bed assuring her it was okay to let go. She was a very special woman who had touched the hearts of both relatives and friends. Many of those people kept vigil, supporting her family and sharing their love for and with her.

My heart was terribly heavy as I sat at her bedside because she was so much more than my patient. She was my dear friend. Stephanie died at 2:00 a.m., Wednesday, with Mike at her side, her daughter Darcy sitting on her bed, and other family and friends about the home. As hard as it was to give her up, it was such a relief to know that the struggle was over for her.

Stephanie, what a privilege to walk the final journey with a very special friend.

## CAREGIVER'S ❁ REFLECTION

### Meditation

Allow God's love to pour into you like sunshine on a spring morning.

Receive this love.

Feel this love renew your spirit.

Visualize this Divine Love uniting you with your loved one.

Be at peace.

### Prayer

Divine Gift-Giver,
you have blessed me
with the treasure of love.

Thank you for the relationship
that I have with my dear one
who is dying.

Even when I am filled with sadness
I will not forget this gift
of beautiful love.

I will savor each moment
I have with my loved one,
no matter how difficult it is,
because I know that love
is uniting us.

## For Today

I will often look upon my loved one with the eyes of
love.

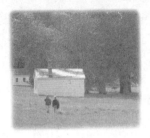

# SIXTEEN

# Everything Must Be Done

I cared for a capable, organized man who had cancer of the esophagus. His daughter contacted me to see him after he made the decision to discontinue chemotherapy. Two courses of chemotherapy had made him quite sick and the tumor had enlarged in spite of it. When I went to see Richard, he didn't think there was much he needed from hospice right away. Although he was tired and often weak, he was not really in pain. He wanted to get a lot done and enumerated the lists of things he just had to do before he died. Richard was pleasant, but also a bit tense and guarded. I made arrangements that day to see him weekly, assuring him that I would visit as often as he needed.

When I saw Richard the next several weeks he kept me posted on the progress of his "to do" list. He had his funeral planned and pall bearers chosen but still needed to write what he wanted said at his funeral. He wanted to do errands, like talking to his banker and contacting a monument company about his gravestone, yet he was feeling a little too unsteady to drive. Richard also missed going to the drugstore and having coffee with the guys like he used to do. We made arrangements for me to take him to do this. I assured him that we would spend the morning of the following week doing his errands. Richard seemed quite happy with the plan and started to warm up to me.

Three days later, I picked him up at 9:00 a.m. and drove him to the drugstore downtown. He had called a few of his buddies to tell them he was coming, and they were anxious to see him. I could tell, as we drove to the drugstore, that even though he was tired and pushing himself, he was excited to be going. I dropped him off with a promise that I would be back in thirty to forty-five minutes to check on him and see how things were going. I waited thirty minutes and went back. He seemed to be enjoying himself so I slipped away quietly, hoping he wouldn't see me and think he should go. Fifteen minutes later I came back just as Richard was getting up from the table. When we got into the car, he sank into the seat. I could tell he was exhausted. He smiled and said, "It was so good to visit with my friends. I could tell they were glad to see me, but now I'm worn out." I took him home, helped him into the house, got him situated in his recliner, and bid him good-bye. He expressed such a genuine "thank-you" that it touched my heart.

The next week when I picked Richard up for his planned list of errands, he was very intent on getting everything done. I drove him to the door of the hardware store where he took a small window screen to be repaired for a bedroom window. In a little while he came out, walking as briskly as he could. He got into the car and was rather short of breath. I explained to him that he didn't need to rush for my sake; I had all morning and I would help him get everything done.

Then we went to see Richard's insurance agent. He took some papers that he had with him and it was apparent that he was a man on a mission. He was in there about thirty minutes. When he came back, I asked, "Where are we going next, Richard?" He said, "Is it okay if we keep going?" I responded, "Sure, as long as you feel like it."

Richard took care of his tasks at the monument company, got back in the car, and asked, "Do you have more time?" I answered, "Sure I do. What next?" He suggested rather apologetically, "I'd like to go to the bank in Story City, which is twenty miles away." "We can do that," I said, and away we went.

All the way to Story City and back Richard talked about his life. He told me how he had been an alcoholic for many years before finally going for treatment. With a proud voice, he described the way he had worked with alcoholics in AA and helped people who were struggling with addictions. Richard spoke about his family, his worries and concerns about dying without everything being in order for them. He reflected on how he had parented, being too strict at times but feeling he had to keep control over his six kids. He spoke with remorse about the way he treated his family when he was drinking and how he hoped they had, or would, forgive him. He also talked a lot about a grandson whom he and Pat had raised and how proud he was of him.

Richard went into the bank in Story City, and when he came out he sounded relieved: "I am so glad I got everything on my list done. Thank you for taking so much time with me." I said, "Richard, there's a little time left. What would you like to do just for fun, or are you tired and needing to go home and rest?" He answered, "I'm very tired, but I don't want to go home just yet. There is one other thing I'd like to do. I have a farm out in the country south of here and I've worked hard through the years to raise Christmas trees. I have a pretty nice crop that my son has taken over. He and his wife live there now, and I'd just like to go see the trees one more time and show them to you."

Away we went, with Richard directing me over the country roads until we came to the farm. The gate was open so I drove into the field of Christmas trees. Richard was quite short of breath by this time and I knew he couldn't walk. I stopped the car and he again reminisced on a deeper level: "I know my life on this earth is about over and I am pretty much ready. I've written my obituary and talked to each one of my kids. I am so glad I have my faith and that I know where I am going. I just wish I could relax and let go instead of thinking of more things that I need to do."

Richard became very tired so I drove him home, assisted him into the house, and helped him lie down. When Richard thanked me for our day together, I was able to tell him that the level of sharing that he had done with me about his thoughts and feelings was a gift, and I promised him that I would continue to walk beside him to his last breath.

He patted my hand, smiled, and dozed off to sleep. As I drove back to the hospice office tears filled my eyes. I truly felt it was a privilege to spend more than half of a day with him. Two days later, his wife called to say that he was extremely confused, had been very belligerent during the night, and that something had to be done. I made some phone calls and the decision was made to admit him to the hospital. Tests revealed probable brain metastasis and his condition rapidly deteriorated over the next four days.

Monday morning when I went up to the hospital hospice room to see Richard, his lungs were congested and he was non-responsive. It was obvious that he was dying. I slipped in and out of his room every couple of hours, took coffee to the family who has gathered in his room, and offered reassurance when appropriate. About 4:00 p.m., I went to see him one more time before I headed home. As I walked toward his bed I could see that he was taking his last few breaths. I called June, his daughter who was a nurse working downstairs, and asked her to come. Richard's family all gathered around his bed and he breathed four or five more slow breaths and stopped. I suddenly realized that there I was, with him for his last breath as I had promised him I would be.

Thank you, Richard, for allowing me to assist you in getting everything done so that you could complete your journey home with peace of mind and heart.

## CAREGIVER'S ❖ REFLECTION

### *Meditation*

Imagine your loved one standing in an open doorway.

See the Holy One waiting to welcome him (her).

Mentally embrace your loved one and bid farewell.

Watch as your loved one walks through the door.

See how he (she) walks into the arms of the Holy One.

Now visualize an angel coming to your side and supporting you.

Receive this kindness and comfort from the angel.

### *Prayer*

Doorway to Home,
my loved one is preparing
for the journey to your eternal dwelling.

May I be attentive to what is needed
and willing to do what I can.
I want to help my loved one
to prepare for the journey Home.

Assist me in listening to the requests,
both hidden and spoken,
that are made by my loved one,
and to do what is possible
in response to these requests.

We are on the journey together.
You will show us the way.
Thank you for your guidance
and your constant, nurturing love.

## *For Today*

---

I will ask my loved one what he (she) needs in
order to prepare for death.

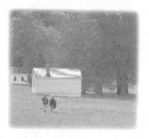

# SEVENTEEN

# A Bit of Heaven on Earth

Tom was a forty-year-old man whom I cared for at the hospice during his last several weeks of life. He had been diagnosed with cancer more than four years earlier and had been through many chemotherapy and radiation treatments. He was married and had three teenage children. Even though he had been very sick, he always thought he would beat the cancer. Tom said he constantly told himself that this treatment or that treatment would be the one that would make him well. He had been in the hospital for a month and was very sick. He was on intravenous pain-medication and was unable to be up much. Although he was extremely ill, Tom still didn't think he would die.

He said that he planned to go back home with the IV and figured he could live a long time, maybe years, on pain medication and other treatments when he needed them. Then he found out his wife couldn't handle his care at home and he thought he would go to a nursing home. He told himself: People live five or ten years in nursing homes. I still am not going to die. Finally, Tom told me, "When they came in and said I was going to this home for hospice patients, I thought: My God, I must be going to die."

I listened intently as Tom continued to describe his process of coming to terms with his dying. "There was no way I wanted to come here. I expected a dark dungeon type of place," he said. "I was quite surprised that it was bright and cheery and that all the people caring for me were happy. After I got admitted, they answered all my questions and took care of my medication. But then, I was alone for the first time. I started really thinking: So I have come here to die. I just really thought about that a lot and I could finally admit it to myself for the first time. After a while, I felt some relief that I didn't have to run from my dying anymore."

One of the nurses had told him that part of the care of hospice is to make every day be the best day it can be. Tom commented, "I started thinking about how that would be." He explained that he had really begun to be aware of how hard it was trying to always run from the thought of dying, to try continually to keep his body stronger than it really was. Then he thought about what dying would be like. He said, "I thought and thought and when my wife and kids came in to visit that evening, I was ready to talk." Tom had them all come around the bed and he told them he had come there because he was going to die. He said he wanted them all to know it so that then they could make whatever time he had left the best that it could be.

Tom seemed at peace. He had a great deal of pain so the pain medication had to be increased to control it. Family and friends visited him daily. His parents from out of state also came often to visit him. They were really struggling with the thought of losing their son and Tom knew that. One morning he requested that instead of the nurse's aide giving him a bath he would like his dad to give him a bath. His dad told us later how scared he was when Tom made that request. He felt very inadequate and wondered: How do I give him a bath? But he said it was a great experience . . . "to give my son a bath and to think I wasn't going to have him on this earth much longer." Tom's dad said that during the bath he recalled days when Tom was a baby and he would help care for him. He cried a lot as he described his experience of giving his forty-year-old son a bath.

Tom told us that he often thought about what heaven would be like. He said he and his family had camped a lot and they loved it. He thought heaven might be like going to a campground. There would be a big campfire and his grandpa who had died would be there. He said he was going to have a beer with grandpa in heaven. As Tom's condition worsened, we asked him if there was anything he would like to do that he had not done. He reminisced about camping and sitting by the campfire and wished that he'd been able to do that one more time.

His parents and his brothers were coming on

Friday and he looked forward to that. On Friday everyone came as planned. Tom was excited. One of the nurses who was caring for him inquired about bringing his bed to the day-room and having a fire in the fireplace there. After some discussion of the "how," furniture was rearranged. We moved Tom (bed, IVs, and all) to the day-room, right in front of a roaring fire, with his wife, children, brothers, parents, and nurses all around him. He had his one last campfire and his loved ones were with him. Tom died several days after this experience.

Thank you, Tom, for allowing me to walk with you as you prepared for your journey to the Great Campground.

CAREGIVER'S ✤ REFLECTION

### Meditation

Picture your loved one with God in a scene that would bring happiness to him (her)

(a campfire, a fishing boat, a beach, a football game, a theater, a library . . . ).

Imagine your loved one enjoying being there.

Send love from your heart to your loved one's heart.

Be at peace.

Eternal Love,
each of us is eventually
called home to you.

Help my loved one
to feel close to you,
to have a hopeful image
of eternity.

May he (she) find courage,
to not run from dying
when the time is near.

Gift my loved one with a strong faith,
to have hope for the future,
and to trust that he (she) will be at peace
when death comes.

## *For Today*

I will rely on my faith to help me to accept the reality
of death.

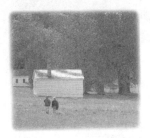

# EIGHTEEN

# The Brass Band Will Play

Jean and her husband, Bob, helped me get a job as a school nurse many years ago when I needed to be home in the summer with my family. It was a time when Gary was first battling cancer and Joe, Mike, and Julie were still young children. With that job I could be home during more of the hours when the kids were home, with weekends and holidays off too.

Now Jean was battling terminal cancer and Bob called to ask if I could come to the hospital to see them. He told me that the doctor had given her more chemotherapy and assured them that Jean was going to be improving soon. Bob said, "That's not what I see. I wish you could help us know what is going on."

I went to the hospital and I could see that Jean was very ill. She was receiving platelet transfusions every day or every other day, and intravenous TPN nutritional feedings. She was very weak, pale, and slightly confused at times. Jean was happy to see me and knew who I was, although she dozed frequently. Bob appeared worn out since he was staying at the hospital all day, every day, and taking turns with the children staying all night. I talked to him more than I did to Jean and supported his frustration—it didn't appear that she would be getting better.

While talking with Bob, he mentioned a family reunion that was coming up on Sunday. I suggested that I stay with Jean so he could go to the reunion. He eagerly accepted the offer. I sat with Jean from 6:00 p.m. to 10:00 p.m. that Sunday. She was more awake than usual and restless at times. She talked about her family, especially about her daughter-in-law who had died of complications of Hodgkin's disease when her children were very small. She was so thrilled that her son, Ben, had remarried and that his new wife, Ann, was such a good mom to the two small children. Jean said that Ann was sent from heaven.

Jean and I also talked about her prognosis and she said she wasn't afraid to die, but she *was* afraid of what she would have to go through before she died. She said that she hated the thought of leaving her family, but then added, "The doctor says I will get better, so we will see." She had pain in her back that night so we got pain medication for her and she was more comfortable then.

A week and a half later, Bob called to say that Jean seemed to be doing worse and the physicians were still talking as if she were about to go home. Bob was tearful and asked if I could come up to the hospital again. I got there within the hour and found Jean sitting in the chair with blood dripping from her mouth. She was slow to respond, very lethargic, and extremely pale. She appeared to be dying. Jean had just received a platelet transfusion, but the bleeding continued. I told Bob I thought he should call his children to come because I believed she had only a short time to live.

Their son came shortly, and he and Bob were sitting on the bed beside Jean's chair. She was very uncomfortable in bed, so the chair became her bed. I sat on the floor and looked up into her eyes because her head was hanging down. I held her hand and said, "Jean, you have fought a hard battle with your cancer and have wanted to be here for Bob and the kids, but you don't have to do that anymore. Jean, it is okay to let go. Bob and the kids will be okay."

Jean said very quietly, "Can I?" I said, "Yes, you can let go. It's okay to go and know that your work on earth is done." She said, "Alleluia." After a bit I said, "You can be there to greet your family when they come to heaven." Jean raised her head a bit, and with a smile she said more loudly, "Then the brass band will play."

Bob and his son were tearful, but also expressed relief and joy. Jean died two days later. As I was greeting the family at her wake, I was surprised when I greeted Ann, the new daughter-in-law whom Jean had liked so much. I recognized Ann immediately. When I saw her, I realized that I had also cared for Ann's dad before he died. As Ann and I talked, she told me that she felt her dad had sent Jean's son and his two children to her.

What miracles there are on this earth and what a privilege it was to assist Jean and her family with the awareness that the end of her life was near. Jean, I hope the brass band played well for you as you walked into eternity.

## CAREGIVER'S ✿ REFLECTION

### *Meditation*

God is a compassionate, loving presence.

When we are experiencing difficulties, God offers tenderness and consolation.

Many times this comfort comes through people around us.

Think today of how God is caring for you and your loved one,

perhaps through hospital or hospice staff, family members, neighbors, pastors or chaplains. . . .

Give thanks for the ways God reaches out to you.

### *Prayer*

Comforting, consoling God,
thank you for those people
who have eased the burdens
of this difficult time of our lives.

Thank you for all those
who have understood the pain
and the many struggles
of my loved one and myself.

Thank you for each one
who has been patient and kind,
for each one who has tried
to ease the hurt and be there for us.

Thank you for being with us
in your many human disguises.

## For Today

I will look for God in the people who are with my
loved one and with myself.

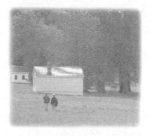

# NINETEEN

# Until Death Do Us Part

Gerald's wife accompanied him when he was admitted to Kavanagh House on a rainy day in March. Gerald had been sick with cancer of the prostate for some time and his wife was no longer able to care for him at home. They shared with us how they had been a team for many years as they took care of and raised their only child, Jack, a son who was born retarded. They had taken care of him in their home his whole life and he was now forty-one years old. Martha had been trying to care for both of them. Finally she and Gerald made the difficult decision to have Gerald enter a hospice facility because she just couldn't handle the care of two of them.

Gerald was lost without Martha. They had been side by side for so many years and it was difficult for him to be without her. He would talk about how lonely he felt when she wasn't there. When she was there to visit with him and left to go home to be with their son, Gerald would wonder when Martha was coming back.

Martha seemed increasingly tired when she came to spend time with Gerald. She talked about not feeling well and how everything took such an effort. As the days passed, we noticed that Martha didn't look well. She was losing weight and her face had a grayish pallor to it. She complained of stomach pain and her abdomen started looking distended. We finally persuaded her (after much encouragement) that she should go to the doctor. She was very reluctant because she felt that she needed to be available to Gerald and to their son. There were two nieces nearby who were able to help out with Jack when Martha had to be admitted to the hospital for tests. There she learned that she had pancreatic cancer and that it was quite extensive.

Martha wanted to go home from the hospital even though we had offered her a place with Gerald at the hospice facility. She continued to feel a great responsibility for Jack and wanted to try to be with him. After just a few days, Martha and her two nieces knew that she could not get the care she needed at home, and we admitted her to the hospice residence where she shared the same room with Gerald. They were both very sick but found much comfort in being side by side, sharing this final stage of their journey just as they had shared so much of the rest of their life's journey.

Even though Martha was initially much sicker than Gerald, he took a turn for the worse after a couple of weeks and, for awhile, we thought he would die soon. This nearness to death prompted them to make a decision about their son's care. Even though they had been greatly concerned about Jack at home, they gradually developed strength and insight about the situation. They realized they had to let go of their responsibility for Jack because they knew they were both dying. Arrangements were made for Jack to go to a group home for adults. Once this was decided, they knew that their work was finished.

We tried to talk to each of them and tell them how the other one was doing. We weren't sure who was going to die first. They seemed somehow to be intensely present to each other even without talking. They had no family to visit them, except for the two nieces who had been so good, helping with Jack and getting him placed in the home.

One evening, Gerald began having periods of apnea and his blood pressure dropped. He was not producing any urine and we knew he was nearing death. We told him it was okay to let go and be free. He had a deep faith and we assured him that God would be there for him and would take his hand when it was time. In a short while, Gerald's breathing stopped. After a bit, the nurse leaned down to Martha's ear and said, "Gerald has gone to heaven, Martha, and he would like you to come along when you can."

Within about five minutes, Martha also quit breathing.

What a miracle—this beautiful couple who had walked their journey of life in step with each other died in step the same way. Thanks, Martha and Gerald, for showing me how to walk the final journey of life together. Your faithful love inspired me.

## CAREGIVER'S ✹ REFLECTION

### *Meditation*

God is a faithful companion. This Source of Strength is always available to you.

Lean your weariness on God's breast today and let God's love comfort you.

You are not alone.

### *Prayer*

Faithful God,
you are with us
every step of the way.

Grant me the capacity to endure
as I give my full attention to my loved one.
I want to be there for him (her)
and do whatever I can.

When it seems I have no strength left,
be my strength and my courage.
When I wonder if I can continue,
fill me with renewed energy.

Thank you for all those who have
stood by me so faithfully.
Thank you for all those
who have encouraged me
and helped me to go on.

Comfort my loved one this day
and give him (her) the grace
of a peaceful journey home.

## For Today

I will thank God for giving me the strength I need.

I will be grateful for those who journey with my
loved one and myself.

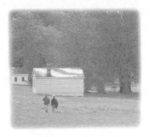

# TWENTY

# Suspicion, Then Trust

Wiley wasn't very interested in help from hospice when we first met. He tended to be private and independent and didn't want much of anything from us. The first time I saw him he denied the fact that he was in pain and experiencing shortness of breath and nausea. He claimed that he was feeling fine, in spite of metastatic lung cancer. When I offered to come see him in a few days, he said he felt no need for me to come for at least a week. I went back the next week, and the following week after that.

The second time I went, I took him a strawberry milkshake. I had discovered he liked these from a previous conversation. I could tell that in spite of his resistance to having much contact with hospice, a friendship was developing between Wiley and me. It wasn't very long after that when he decided it would be good for me to come two or three times a week.

Wiley began talking more, and the visit that cemented our friendship was the day when I asked him to tell me about his wife, who had died six months before I met him.

Wiley talked for an hour about his wife and cried a lot in spite of himself. He described how they had worked together in his business, delivering motor homes and trailer houses from California to anywhere in the United States. He emphasized that they were not only partners in work and marriage, but best friends as well.

During the next several weeks, Wiley was able to share his feelings, fears, and awareness of his declining condition. He lived in a second-floor apartment and his elderly sister, who lived down the hall, had tried to do some cooking and some laundry for Wiley when she recognized his difficult situation. Wiley was becoming much weaker and unsteady on his feet. He even admitted to me that he had fallen one night when getting up to go to the bathroom.

I was fearful about suggesting the possibility of a nursing home placement to Wiley, but I decided I had to be honest and straightforward. I explained to him that I was concerned about his safety and informed him about a hospice room that we had at the local nursing home. He quickly voiced interest in moving and seemed to trust my judgment. That very day I went down the hall and invited his sister to be a part of this conversation so she could hear him express his desire to move. She seemed relieved, and we made the necessary phone calls; he was able to move later that day. I promised Wiley that I would accompany him there, which I did, and the transition went smoothly. He didn't seem to have strong feelings about leaving his apartment, although his sister was very sad.

Wiley lived only eleven days in the nursing home, but he was content there. His condition rapidly deteriorated during the last week with shortness of breath and increasing pain. He became very weak, but he still insisted on spending most of the day in the chair. I went to see him each day, and a few days before he died he said to me, "I'm getting close, aren't I?"

I said, "That's how it seems to me, Wiley. Is that how you feel?" He said, "Yes, and I wish it could be over. Can't you just shoot me? I'm no good anymore." I said, "No, Wiley, I can't shoot you, but I *can* and will continue to walk beside you and make sure you don't have pain and are as comfortable as you choose to be." I also told him that it was okay to let go when he was ready and I wondered aloud if his wife wouldn't be there waiting for him. He smiled, and after a brief pause, said, "I'm sure she is."

Wiley told me he had never gone to church and that he didn't know what would happen to him when he died. He had always declined a chaplain visit and had requested that I not let "all those people" hang around him in the nursing home. I had assured him that it would be like his home and only those people whom he wanted would be allowed in his room. At that moment, he was talking with me like he would with a chaplain, telling me he knew his wife was waiting for him and that he felt peaceful and ready to die. I told Wiley I was happy that he felt that way. After a while, I was just sitting with him and he turned toward me and whispered, "Thanks a lot for all you have done. I love you."

Thank you, Wiley, for giving me a chance to walk beside you and for trusting me as you journeyed home.

## CAREGIVER'S ❈ REFLECTION

### *Meditation*

Think about Jesus and how much he respected the ill and hurting ones.

Picture him with his outstretched hand, touching the sick.

Now, imagine that Jesus reaches out and touches both you and your loved one.

Receive the loving touch of Jesus with hope and with gratitude.

### *Prayer*

Kind and gracious God,
help me to listen attentively
to the thoughts and feelings
of my loved one.

Do not allow my agenda
to dominate his (her) journey.

Help my focus to remain
on what is best for him (her).

Thank you for always approaching me
with dignity and respect.
I pray that I can do the same
with my loved one.

I entrust him (her)
into your hands once again.
Wrap your gracious love around us
and touch us with your care.

## For Today

---

I will accept my loved one and not require that he
(she) meet my expectations.

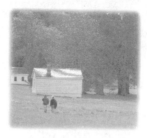

# TWENTY-ONE

# Afraid to Die

My mother was diagnosed with a rare malignant tumor. She died one year later on January 18. Her condition was worsening eight months after diagnosis, and it was obvious that she had, at most, months to live. I went to see her each weekend. She lived seventy miles away, so I would go on Friday after work and come home on Sunday night. My dad did a great job of helping her during the week and I would clean, do laundry, and just be with them on the weekends.

One Friday night, she seemed much different, "very down in the dumps," discouraged, and sad. She had been talkative, realistic, and seemed peaceful prior to this time. I thought maybe Friday had simply been a bad day, so I tried to help her in every way that I could and just be with her in a compassionate way. Dad even seemed more tense, I think because Mother was so discouraged. I felt worried and concerned about Mother's mood.

Saturday morning, I got the house cleaned and the laundry done and encouraged Mom to eat a little breakfast and lunch. I asked Mother once in awhile, "Is something wrong? You seem down this weekend." She would answer me each time, "No, I'm okay." She was getting oxygen continuously. I knew she had a doctor's appointment on Tuesday and would probably have to have some fluid taken from her lung, a thoracentesis, which she was having to have done every three weeks or so. I asked her if she was dreading going to the doctor on Tuesday and she said, "No." I inquired if she was having any pain and she also said "no" to that question. She continued to be quiet, withdrawn, and didn't make much eye contact with me.

My mother and I had had conflicts in our relationship at times prior to her diagnosis of cancer. She was often displeased with me because she thought that I didn't care about her enough, and I always felt I couldn't do anything right when I was around her. After her diagnosis of cancer, our relationship was better. It seemed that now, when she finally had the illness that she had always dreaded, she could focus on it. In turn, her illness gave me a direction in which I could specifically extend my love. I knew how to take care of her and meet her needs.

I also knew my mother was going to die and the small conflicts that used to get in our way didn't matter anymore. She loved how I cared for her and fussed over her and I loved doing it. I had always longed to have her know how much I truly cared about her. This particular weekend, however, she was very depressed and didn't respond to anything. I was worried by her change of mood, but no matter which way I asked her about how she was feeling or what was bothering her, she denied anything was wrong.

Sunday morning came and I was getting frantic. I didn't think I could go back home and leave her this way. I didn't know what to do. Mid-morning Sunday I went into the living room and sat down beside Mother. I just sat with her a while and then I took her hand and looked into her eyes. I said, "Mother, please tell me what is bothering you. I know something is wrong and I want you to share your unhappiness with me if you can. I will do anything to help you if you will just tell me what you are so down about."

After a while she started crying and large tears rolled down her face. Pretty soon she said to me, "I know I'm going to die and I think I'm going to go to hell because I've made mistakes in my life." Then she cried some more. I felt helpless because I knew she wasn't going to hell, but I didn't know how to talk to her about it. I said a little prayer to myself that I would find the right words to convince her otherwise. I asked her why she thought she was going to go to hell and she repeated her reason: she had made lots of mistakes in her life and didn't think she was a very good wife or mother. I assured her, "Mother, you are not going to hell."

I asked her if she felt she had done the best that

she could at being a wife and mother and she eagerly said, "Oh yes, I did the very best that I knew how." I then explained to her that the God that I believed in was a loving God, not a critical God, and I was convinced that God made her just the way that he wanted Madelyn LaFollette to be—knowing that she could only try to give her best. I assured her that it was human to make mistakes, that God continues to love us, forgive us, and allow us to learn from our mistakes.

She then reminisced about some things that caused her to feel guilty. She explained to me that she always thought that we had to be perfect to go to heaven. I again talked about God's love for us and I reminded her of her unfailing love and sacrifice for her husband and five children, her kindness to her neighbors and friends, and the way she cared for her own mother in her home when she was dying of cancer. I assured her over and over that she had lived by the greatest commandment given to us: "Love one another."

At the end of a very long afternoon, after lengthy conversation and prayer together, she said to me, "I hope you are right." She cried again and I held her, assuring her that God loved her very much and that her mother and her son (my twin brother, Joe) would be there waiting for her when her time came to die. Before I left that Sunday night, Mom said to me, "I think I do have hope now that I will go to heaven. It's nice to think that I have done the best I could with my life. I don't feel so scared anymore."

Mom, thanks for sharing that part of your journey

with me. Thank you for allowing me to help convince you how very much you were loved by God. You also allowed me to know how very much I love you. Walking you home was another wonderful gift of love that you gave to me.

## CAREGIVER'S ✸ REFLECTION

### *Meditation*

Picture God as a kind and merciful being.

Rest in this peace and let it fill your soul.

See God waiting with open arms for your loved one.

God smiles and says, "Welcome home!"

Imagine all guilt, fear, and concern leaving his (her) spirit.

Carry this peace to your loved one today.

### *Prayer*

Merciful and welcoming Spirit,
you await the arrival of my loved one.

Send your angel of peace
to dissolve any guilt and concern
about past grievances and failures.
May he (she) be convinced
of your unconditional love.

May I be attentive and aware
of any inner distress that my loved one
may be experiencing.

Help me to be kind, reassuring,
and affirming.
May my nonjudgmental attitude
allow him (her) to speak about
anything that is distressful.

## For Today

I will do what I can to bring peace of mind and
heart to my loved one.

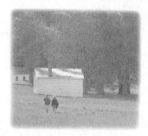

# TWENTY-TWO

# Going Toward the Light

Linda was a thirty-eight-year-old woman whom I took care of several years ago. She had metastatic cancer and had been battling it for four years. She was very sick when I first met her, weak and pain-filled. We were able to get her on medication and this helped to get her pain under control, but her weakness rapidly became worse.

Linda told me that she had three almost-grown children and an eight-year-old boy. She was a single parent and had a very difficult marriage that had ended five years before. She felt okay about the three older children, and with the help of her parents and other relatives and friends, she was pretty confident that they would get along okay. This was not the case, however, with Zachary, the eight-year-old. She was desperate not to die because she knew Zachary needed her.

Soon after I started caring for her, she was telling me about her life and her family, and she shared her fear of dying and leaving Zachary with no parent. She said, "I know the doctor says there is nothing more to do to stop the cancer from growing, but I absolutely cannot die." She said, occasionally, with great determination, "I have to figure my way out of this. I am not going to die." Linda became more active for a time because we were able to control her pain. She could function better and therefore decided that maybe she could "beat the cancer."

She had lots of company—family and friends were willing to help and wanted to take some of the burden and worries from Linda. She was open about suggesting what they might do to relieve her of her responsibilities—all except Zachary. She felt guilty that he had only had a father in his life for a little while and, now, would not have a mother either. She would say things like, "I shouldn't have brought him into this world if I couldn't take care of him. This is all so unfair to him."

She started getting weaker and more short of breath. As she felt her condition worsening, she verbalized more strongly, "I am not going to die. I've got to figure my way out of this. I can't leave Zachary."

Early on a Thursday morning, when I went to care for Linda, she appeared to be actively dying. Several days before we had started a continuous IV morphine drip because her pain had become uncontrollable with the oral morphine. Her eyes were glassy and had a far away look. Her breathing was labored and moist. Her skin was cool to the touch and starting to look mottled at her knees and ankles. She was only slightly responsive verbally but was able to hear what I said to her and could let me know that she heard me.

I spent the day with Linda, talking to her about what was going on, increasing her pain medication when she would indicate to me that she was hurting. She was receiving oxygen continuously through a nasal cannula. She would sleep for a time and then she would tense her muscles and try to sit up, but was too weak to do so. She would yell Zachary's name. When she did so, I would talk into her ear, telling her that her family and friends would keep Zachary safe and take care of him, as they promised they would.

I spoke to her softly about the fact that she was probably dying and that some patients had told me about a light that they saw when they were dying. It was full of love and it was so peaceful to go to that light. It was full of love just for them. I said, "Linda, if you see a light, why don't you go toward it because it will be full of love for you."

Every time she jerked her body and tried to sit up and yell for Zachary, I would tell her I was with her and that I was going to keep staying beside her. I continually urged her: "Breathe deeply. Try to relax." I kept assuring her that she was doing well. I spoke softly into her ear to tell her what was going on. It felt very much like being beside a woman in labor who was about to give birth, except the labor now was that of giving birth to new life beyond this earthly one.

This woman in the throes of the labor of dying would relax and sleep for a time and then would tense up and go through some contraction type of movement while calling her son's name. Each time became longer apart and less intense—she seemed to be more relaxed. I would frequently tell her I was with her and that she was doing well, that everyone was going to be okay, and that she could let go whenever she chose. Her parents sat in the waiting room across the hall and would only come to her side for short periods of time. They said that was as much as they could endure.

Then Linda's breathing became very shallow. I whispered into her ear: "Go on, Linda, you are almost there. Just let go when you want and go to peace and love." She became very relaxed with a peaceful and serene expression on her face. She took a few more breaths and then died.

Thank you, Linda, for allowing me to be your birthing coach as you experienced the labor pains of your journey home.

## CAREGIVER'S 🎇 REFLECTION

### Meditation

Light a candle. Sit by the candle in silence for awhile.

Then, visualize the Divine Presence as a beautiful sphere of light.

Let this Light surround you and fill you with serenity.

Rest in the goodness and comfort of this Great Light.

Birthing God,
you accompany us into this world
and you journey with us
into the next.

Come, with your loving voice
and urge my loved one to come home.
Console, encourage, and comfort him (her).

Enkindle the hearts of all of us
who walk with this loved one.

O Divine Light,
draw this loved one home,
to the radiance of your love.

*For Today*

I will be aware of all external forms of light as reminders of the Great Light who draws the dying to their eternal home.

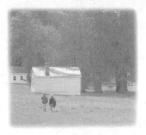

# TWENTY-THREE

# Intimate Love—Intimate Death

I once met a delightful couple who were sad, disappointed, and extremely perplexed by the journey that was suddenly thrust upon them. You see, Galen and Claudia were very much in love and had only been married for two months. They had met a couple of years earlier. She was a divorcée with three teenage children, he had never been married.

About a year before I met them, Galen admitted to Claudia that he did not feel well at times. He was hesitant to tell her because his religious belief did not allow medical intervention. His religion told him to control it with the mind, to take care of it within himself and with God. This seemed to work pretty well initially. Claudia tried very hard to believe with him, but because it wasn't her belief of origin, she was sometimes scared and distrustful. Anyway, they decided to be married and were very excited as they made wedding plans. Her three children loved Galen. He fit into their family as if he had always been there. They had a wonderful wedding with family and friends gathered around them.

They treasured their time together and Claudia could hardly believe anyone could be so good to her after her past experience with marriage. Life was nearly perfect. They went to Hawaii for their honeymoon, but Galen became quite ill while they were there. He contacted a minister of his religion in Hawaii. They prayed, read scripture together, and Galen again believed he could overcome his illness. Medical intervention still was not an alternative for him. Claudia, who was losing hope, continued to stand beside him although she longed for him to seek medical help.

When they returned home they tried to start marriage at a normal pace. Their love was strong and they believed they could overcomes Galen's illness and that he would be okay. Several weeks later, Galen became so ill and full of pain that Claudia took him to the emergency room. He was admitted to the hospital and, after a few days of tests, was found to have extensive cancer, with a prognosis of "days to a few weeks" to live. The cancer was so widespread that radiation or chemotherapy was not an option, nor would his belief system have allowed for those treatments.

Galen was transferred to a hospice facility for symptom management and care. This is when I first met this incredible couple who were so in love. By this time, Galen was extremely ill, and it did not appear initially that he had more than a few days to live. He was obviously experiencing inner turmoil because of some guilt over his decision not to seek medical treatment, particularly for pain control. It was also obvious from our first encounter that if love could cure him, he would be alive and well in a day or two.

This so-in-love couple were desperately sad. Galen was unable to let go of believing that, if he just believed enough and had enough faith, he still would be able to bring his devastating disease under control. At the same time, he became increasingly aware that he was quickly losing ground. Claudia was overcome with conflict and sadness as she processed her anger and resentment about his belief system, the system that had denied him any medical treatment early on. Her overwhelming love for this man increased her heartache as she watched him die in front of her eyes.

When they celebrated their two month anniversary at the hospice facility, the staff quickly decorated Galen's room with a bed and breakfast atmosphere for the special day. They even put a privacy sign on the door. Galen and Claudia were able to share their love in their own way on their anniversary. They used part of the day to make a tape recording on which they expressed their love for each other.

As Galen neared the time of his death, Claudia recognized intellectually that it was happening and was able to give him permission to die even though her heart felt shattered in a million pieces. When Galen died a week later, Claudia spoke of the two month anniversary as one of their times together that she would always cherish in memory.

Dying is a very intimate experience, as intimate as a two-month wedding anniversary. Thank you, Galen and Claudia, for allowing me to walk beside you at the end of that most intimate of journeys.

## CAREGIVER'S ❧ REFLECTION

### *Meditation*

Sit quietly. Remember that God is with you.

Open your heart to receive God's all-embracing love for you.

Let these words sink into your mind and heart:

"Love is stronger than death" (Song of Songs 8:6).

Bring this truth into your whole being.

Let it give you comfort and strength.

### *Prayer*

Beloved God,
you have embraced us
with a love that endures all things.

The power of your unending love
will see us through the times
when we feel empty and bereft.

When the days are long and desolate
draw us to your heart,
strengthen us, and comfort us.
Reassure us that the love we share
with one another
will go on into eternity.

Beloved God,
thank you for love
that is stronger than death.

## *For Today*

---

I will remember that love is stronger than death.

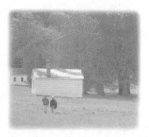

# TWENTY-FOUR

# The End of the Road

A home care agency called me to see a patient of theirs who had been with them for quite awhile. His condition was deteriorating and they had been unable to adequately relieve the constant pain he had had for several months. They told me that this man was very depressed and seemed to have no will to live anymore.

I called his home and made an appointment to see him and his wife the next day. I went on a cloudy, rainy day and the house looked dark and dismal as I entered. Don and Betty were sitting at the kitchen table eating a meager lunch. The small house was clean and arranged to meet their needs, with a daybed in the corner of the dining room where Betty slept. They had not been able to sleep together for a long time because she had severe osteoporosis and wore a body brace. She suffered quietly and bravely and all her concern was focused on her dying husband. Betty repeated what the home care agency had told me and added that Don had been getting very forgetful the past several months and was confused at times, especially at night.

Soon after I arrived, Don very feebly made his way to the living room with the help of his walker and sat down in his chair. Betty trailed behind him with another walker, although she stood beside his chair instead of sitting down. When I offered to put a chair beside him for her, she explained that she was more comfortable standing, leaning on her walker. Sitting caused her discomfort.

I sat down and explained that Andrea, their home care nurse, had asked me to come and tell them about hospice services because she felt Don could benefit from it. After I described hospice care to them, we then discussed the constant pain that he was having. I assured him that comfort was our priority and that I was confident that we could help him after assessing his situation. I learned that the pain medication had not been taking his pain away because he had been forgetting to take it.

Don was very thin and sat in his chair most of the time, using oxygen for his shortness of breath. Because of his being in the chair so much, he also had an open sore on his coccyx. I called the doctor and got the pain medication changed to a patch to be put on the skin. It would give him a steady dose of pain medication and they wouldn't have to get up so often in the night to take medication. Don also had not taken the pain medication at times because he became constipated and knew that the pain medication caused it. Putting him on a laxative/stool softener program took care of that problem.

After I had explained everything to them, Don and Betty both verbalized their relief at having hospice. Then I asked Don, "What does having hospice mean to you? What does it feel like?" He was quiet for awhile and then he looked into my face and said very quietly, "It's like having two bullets left in the gun. It's the end of the road." He and Betty were tearful for a time, and so was I. It was pretty clear to me, from my evaluation of him, that Don didn't have long to live.

I made arrangements to come back the next day in case they had questions and to see how his comfort level was. Don was dozing in his chair when I arrived, but Betty was awake. She again expressed her gratitude for hospice and said she hoped Don wouldn't have to linger a long time. The next day, he was more comfortable but very drowsy, and Betty reported that he was eating very little. He had slept most of the night and had not awakened with pain as he usually did.

Three days later, Don got up in the middle of the night to go to the bathroom and fell. Betty couldn't do a thing to get him up. She called 911 and he was taken to the hospital. He was confused, very weak, and moaned continually. An IV of continuous morphine was started and he was admitted to the hospice room of the hospital. Betty was so tired and uncomfortable that she didn't go to the hospital with him. His son who lived close by was at the hospital when the ambulance arrived. I called Betty the next morning when I knew it was her breakfast time and asked her if she would like me to bring her to the hospital. When I went to pick her up, she expressed her dread about riding in a car to go anywhere because her bones broke so easily. She worried about even a small bump in the road so I drove the four blocks to the hospital extra slowly and cautiously.

It was obvious when we arrived that Don was dying. I had learned from my previous visits with them that they were very private people, so I left them alone and after a time I returned with some coffee for Betty. She was sitting beside the bed on the edge of a folding chair, holding his hand, and he was sleeping, breathing heavily, with the oxygen bottle bubbling in the background. After a bit of time, she said to me, "I've told Don it's okay to go and I've said my good-bye. I need to go home now. I can't stay any longer."

When I took Betty home I could tell her heart was heavy. She was concerned that it might appear she didn't care enough about Don, but she said she had to go lie down in her bed. I assured her that if she wanted to come back to the hospital in the afternoon either I, or a volunteer, would come for her. If she chose not to come back, that was okay too.

I went back to the hospital after I took Betty home and Don died shortly after I arrived. The social worker and I called their son and then went home to tell Betty of his death. She said she knew he was going to die soon, but she just couldn't stay to be with him. She was tearful, but also relieved that it was over for him.

There was something I observed during the times I spent with this couple and I asked Betty if I could share it with her. I then told her that in all my years of hospice care I had never observed the kind of gentle patience and affirmation that she displayed as she frequently stood leaning on her walker beside Don's chair, waiting to hear him try to tell a story, lose his thought, become frustrated, and sometimes trail off to a different subject. She would kindly remind him of what he wanted to say, always giving him the opportunity and time to try to remember. She would very lovingly look into his face with a powerful demonstration of acceptance and understanding.

Thank you, Don and Betty, for allowing me to accompany you on Don's final journey home and for teaching me about unconditional love.

## CAREGIVER'S ❊ REFLECTION

### *Meditation*

Sit in a chair that is comfortable for you.

Picture God sitting next to you.

Feel how present God is to you, how caring, how patient.

God does not expect anything from you.

You need only sit and have God as your faithful companion.

Sit for as long as you can.

Give thanks to this tender Companion for being so near.

## *Prayer*

Vigilant Companion,
your steady and faithful presence
is always with me.

You are here as I care for my loved one.
You will be here when my loved one dies.

When I feel helpless,
when all I can do is watch and wait,
gentle me with your patience and kindness.

Help me to affirm my loved one,
to offer understanding and appreciation
of who he (she) is.

May my caring presence
enable him (her) to find a ray of love
in each new day, in each passing hour.

May I be as accepting of my loved one
as you always are of me.

## *For Today*

I will keep vigil with loving patience and kindness.

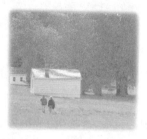

# TWENTY-FIVE

# The Power of Prayer

Catherine was an acquaintance whom I had known for many years. When she was diagnosed with cancer of the colon four years before she died, she had a lot of hope that chemotherapy and radiation would get rid of any cancer that might be left behind after surgery. She did well for about a year, and then it became apparent that there was progression of the disease. Her treatment was changed and she was still able to function well, but she lost her strong sense of hope that she would "beat the cancer."

Faith was always very important in Catherine's life and she believed in the power of prayer. Although she worked part-time outside the home, her central focus of life was on raising her four sons and being a strong marriage partner. Her youngest son, Anthony, was in college when she was diagnosed and by that time she had three grandchildren who were also her pride and joy.

Catherine was very active in her church and became a sponsor for a woman taking classes in preparation for joining her church. Attending those classes gave Catherine a fresh and different viewpoint of her faith. She said that for the first time she realized that things weren't just black and white and that she needed to search, study, and meditate in order to deepen her faith life. The "spiritual side of life" became even more important for Catherine after these classes and gave her an increased inner power that sustained her in the rough times to come. She accepted her spirituality as a natural part of her life and was open and willing to share her beliefs with anyone who asked her about them.

Initially, Catherine believed that prayer would bring a cure for her or that she would, at least, have a long time to live. As her disease progressed, however, she realized that what was important was not how much time she had but, rather, what she did with the time that was left for her to live. She told me one evening that even though prayer had not inspired a cure, the setbacks had not stifled her faith. She was concerned for her husband, Steve, as he struggled with what the future would bring, and she hoped that her prayer would strengthen him.

Catherine's condition plateaued for a time and then slowly deteriorated. Because she was unable to take enough oral nourishment to survive, a decision was made to install a permanent type of intravenous line so she could be fed daily nutrition. This was not an easy procedure to live with, but Catherine seldom complained.

At the same time, her husband became very ill with severe pancreatitis and he, too, had a very guarded prognosis for awhile. Steve spent several days in the intensive care unit and was in the hospital almost three months. During this time, Catherine's inner strength again carried her through as she was at his side each day offering her support and compassion, believing they would get through it together. Everyone was amazed at the way she functioned, putting her own needs aside to be the supportive person she had always been in their relationship. Steve recovered, returned home, and life then centered around long rest periods for each of them.

Not long after Steve came home, their eldest son, Brian, was in a car accident and was rushed to the hospital's intensive care unit. Catherine and Steve were at his side and, again, Catherine's spiritual strength and faith helped to sustain them as they kept vigil with Brian and prayed for his healing.

Brian recovered, but Catherine was becoming aware that her time on this earth was limited. She was concerned with how Steve would cope after she was gone and she encouraged him to talk to a counselor about how to prepare for life without her. She prayed often for him because she knew he was desperate for her to survive and that he feared he couldn't live without her. After months of counseling, he was able to accept the reality of Catherine's approaching death. During conversations they had about how Steve might cope after she died, Catherine always encouraged him to rely on his faith and on prayer for strength and guidance.

Catherine experienced much pain as the disease progressed, and pain medications frequently had to be increased to keep her comfortable. As usual, though, she seldom complained and would often find peace in offering her pain as a way to make herself stronger. Finally, the pain was so intense that during the last weeks of her life, Catherine had to be hospitalized for IV pain medication. Even during her dying she continued to be focused on the needs of her family, committed to being a wife and mother, constantly inquiring how each one was doing. She even arranged a time to be with each one individually, to give them a time to talk with her and to say some cherished things to them before she died.

The power of prayer in Catherine's life was the driving force and the nourishment that gave her the strength to continue her role of wife and mother throughout her illness. Thank you, Catherine, for your powerful example of faith and your commitment to your family as you journeyed home.

## CAREGIVER'S REFLECTION

### *Meditation*

"Come to me, all you that are weary,
and are carrying heavy burdens,
and I will give you rest" (Matthew 11:28).

Picture yourself being held in the arms of God.

Feel the comfort and reassurance that God offers you.

Let go and rest in God's embrace.

## *Prayer*

Shepherd of Souls,
you promise me rest and consolation.
I come to you,
knowing how much I need you
in my life.

You know the longings
of my heart,
even if I cannot find the words
to speak to you.

When I am too tired to pray,
assure me that you hold me close
and that you understand.

I bring my loved one to you.
Grant him (her) whatever is needed
for the journey home to you.

I also bring myself to you.
Grant that I never stop believing
in the power of prayer
and in the strength of your love.

## *For Today*

I will unite my heart with the heart of God and
receive the strength I need.

It was Easter Sunday morning when Joyce Hutchison walked into church and slipped into an already over-crowded pew. She was surprised at how full the church already was, fifteen minutes before Mass was sched-uled to begin. As she casually glanced around her, her heart leaped. There, next to her was the husband and two daughters of Stephanie, the nurse who had died of sinus cancer (story #15). The two girls had been two and five years old when their mother died and now, there they were, aged eleven and fourteen, looking radiant in their Easter finery, seemingly happy and enjoying life. Stephanie's husband recognized Joyce and greeted her warmly, but the girls had been too young to remember her very well, so Joyce re-introduced herself to them and explained how she had known them.

After Mass the reminiscing began. Joyce asked the girls what they remembered about their mother and they, in turn, listened as she told them beautiful stories of Stephanie and described the special friendship they had shared. Joyce couldn't believe how much Darcy, the fourteen-year-old, looked just like her mother. When she remarked about this, Darcy replied proudly that everyone told her about the resemblance and that she loved it because she knew how much people had enjoyed her mother.

Joyce called me later that day and told me about her wonderful Easter experience. We both thought that it was especially remarkable because it happened dur-ing the week when we were completing work on this book. When I heard the story, I couldn't help thinking how it was a reminder of the hope that we want to convey to caregivers who read and use this book.

We know that being a caregiver for someone who is very ill can be a tremendously challenging and draining process. No matter how much we love someone or how responsible we feel about caring for that person, the role of caregiver can often consume one's life and leave little time and energy for anything else. In some cases, caregivers have been offering support and help for such a long time that they have almost forgotten what life was like before they were involved in the caregiver's role. While there may be a sense of peace in the caregiving process, usually there is a tremendous amount of daily adjustment, worry, strain, and distress.

There is simply no way that we can convince anyone that his or her life will be happy again when he or she is in the throes of caring for a loved one who is dying. However, as Joyce said so well, "Seeing Stephanie's family at Mass on Easter Sunday was such a powerful moment for me. It renewed my belief that not only does life go on after a loved one dies, but life can eventually unfold with joy and beauty, even though the loss of a loved one is always a reality in our lives."

And so we say to you, "Do not give up. Hold hope in your heart. Give of your time, energy, and love to those who are on their way home. As you walk with them, keep holding a strong piece of hope deep within your heart. You are walking through the valley to the other side. You can find joy again. You can be at peace."

—JOYCE RUPP

# Leave-Taking

BY SANDRA BURY

*(When death begins to call)*

When the coming of your death
became an awareness on the planet
some wondrous events began.
The word went out that you were preparing
   to leave,
to leave this place that you call home.

The word was heard by the wind
and it promised to blow
under you and push you.

The clouds heard the wind and
billowed for joy.
"You may land on us and float for a while."

The rain said, "I'll wash the air clean,"
while each star polished itself to a
brilliant shine.

In the presence of your impending death
the earth prepared to send you forth.
The gravity that had held you so tightly
began to lose its grip.
It called, "Let loose, Let loose,
Let loose and fly."

As you began to float, a squirrel
noticed and remembered;
remembered how you saved,
saved those things that were important.

He told the rabbit, who told the turtle, who
    told the bird.
"He/She's coming," they whispered.
The bird sang your memories a joyous release.
The song was heard by a lone wolf.

The lone wolf stood on a cold tundra
howling her appreciation of all the
lessons you learned so well.

Some distant great pines heard the howl
    and knew of your leaving.
They swayed, releasing their fragrance
    to waft with you.

The fragrance was gathered in
by the swiftest of hawks, flown high
with the wisdom that the great hawk knows.

The hawk told a passing eagle who
    swooped and soared until,
finding your spirit loose on the wind,
carried it forward to a joyous rainbow.

The rainbow said, "Come, I've been waiting.
The colors are all for you!"

When the moon heard this, it shouted,
"Prepare! A life well lived is approaching!"

The stars again polished their shine
until the illumination penetrated the system.

Your soul saw and knew it was going home.
Home to the light, home to the sun and home
beyond home, beyond home.

And it met with all that it had always known:
the silent and brilliant mystery.
The source.

The entire mystery burst with the splendor of
"welcome, welcome, we have been waiting."
The source, with all the ancestors gathered
    round,
enfolded you and danced your coming.

While far away, in the world you had known,
a group of your loves and friends
gathered to speak your praises,
to sing your leaving and
to forever remember.

JOYCE RUPP, O.S.M., is well known for her work as a writer, spiritual "midwife," and retreat and conference speaker. A member of the Servite (Servants of Mary) community, she has led retreats throughout North America, as well as in Europe, Asia, and Africa. Joyce is the author of many articles and seven books, among them *The Cup of Our Life* and *May I Have This Dance*, (from Ave Maria Press) and *Dear Heart Come Home* (from Crossroad Publishing).

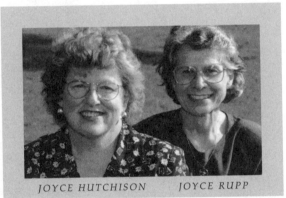

*JOYCE HUTCHISON    JOYCE RUPP*

Photo credit: Chuck Carpenter

JOYCE HUTCHISON, R.N., C.R.N.H., currently serves as Patient Advocate at Mercy Hospital Medical Center in Des Moines, Iowa. Her clinical experience includes work as an oncology nurse, home care nurse, and residence team director of a hospice facility. A member of the National Hospice Organization and the Oncology Nursing Society, she is a frequent presenter of workshops on care of the dying and hospice care.